WALK IT OFF!

20 MINUTES A DAY TO HEALTH AND FITNESS

DR. SUZANNE LEVINE

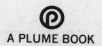

A PLUME BOOK

PLUME
Published by the Penguin Group
Penguin Books USA Inc., 375 Hudson Street,
New York, New York 10014, U.S.A.
Penguin Books Ltd, 27 Wrights Lane,
London W8 5TZ, England
Penguin Books Australia Ltd, Ringwood,
Victoria, Australia
Penguin Books Canada Ltd, 2801 John Street,
Markham, Ontario, Canada L3R 1B4
Penguin Books (N.Z.) Ltd, 182–190 Wairau Road,
Auckland 10, New Zealand

Penguin Books Ltd, Registered Offices:
Harmondsworth, Middlesex, England

First published by Plume, an imprint of New American Library, a division of Penguin
Books USA Inc.

First Printing, December, 1990
10 9 8 7

Ⓟ REGISTERED TRADEMARK—MARCA REGISTRADA

Library of Congress Cataloging-in-Publication Data

Levine, Suzanne M.
    Walk it off! : 20 minutes a day to health and fitness / by
Suzanne M. Levine.
        p. cm.
    ISBN 0-452-26535-5
    1. Physical fitness. 2. Walking—Health aspects. I. Title.
GV481.L58   1991
613.7′1—dc20   90-41033
                                                         CIP

PRINTED IN THE UNITED STATES OF AMERICA
Set in Times Roman
Designed by Leonard Telesca

Contents

Acknowledgments   vii

Introduction   1

PART ① GETTING STARTED   7

1 Walking and You   9
2 Walking Readiness   23
3 The Happy Walker   38

PART ② BUILDING A WALKING HABIT   59

4 The Facts   61
5 The Feelings   70
6 The Rewards   89

PART ③ ON THE ROAD   103

7 Choosing Shoes for Walking   105
8 What to Wear in Any Weather   114
9 Where to Walk Safely   127

PART ④ THE WALKER'S DIET   139

10 The Happy Eater   141

11   Eating and You   159

PART 5   **THE HEALTHY WALKER   189**

12   Pampering Your Feet   191
13   Questions and Answers About Walking and Health   204

PART 6   **ADVANCED WALKING   217**

14   Games People Play While Walking   219
15   Walking Plus: Adding Other Exercises   228
16   Preventing Relapses   240

The Walker's Log   253

Acknowledgments

This book was made possible by the support and help of a key group of people. Editorial consultant and writer Ronni Sandroff helped shape the Walk It Off! program and the concept of this volume. My editor, Alexia Dorszynski, encouraged me to let my personal story unblushingly unfurl in these pages.

Many thanks to Ronni Sandroff, and to Brown Shoe Co. for giving me the opportunity to speak to audiences throughout the U.S. about walking. I owe much to the support of my loyal office crew: Dr. Joann Bilello, Lila Nadel, Dr. John Connors, Rachel Elkayam, and Nancy Sparrow. And a salute, too, to my family: my parents, Miriam and Maurice Marin, my husband, Bart, and my daughters, Marisa and Heather, for putting up with my traveling and appetite for challenge.

I'd like to dedicate this book to all those readers who are in search of a better self-image and a healthier daily routine. Happy walking!

WALK IT OFF!

Introduction

This book is for the rest of us—the 66 percent of all Americans who have resisted the fitness craze. Throughout the late 1970s and the 1980s the news was dominated by exercise images, from the lone runner in the rain to throngs of people panting through marathons and triathlons. The latest exercise machines and rows of bouncing aerobic dancers were flashed before our eyes. "No gain without pain" was a national slogan. A good many people, about a third of the American population, joined the fitness movement and began to exercise vigorously and regularly. But many of the rest of us gave it a brief try and then said, "That's not for me."

If you're in the latter group, this book is for you. I wrote it for the health-club dropout, the exercise-injured, and all those who *hate* to exercise. To put it another way, I wrote the book for people like me. Although I now actually relish my daily walk, until a few years ago I thought I'd never escape my upbringing.

I was a born-and-raised couch potato. Both my parents are heavy-set, sedentary people. As a child, I was encouraged to read, paint, and study hard, but never to dance, play ball, or ride a bike. I was not only a chubby little girl, I had a foot problem and wore clunky orthopedic shoes that made it impossible to skip, jump, or run. Even when our family went to the beach, we lounged on the blanket eating and reading, while other families cavorted in the waves and threw Frisbees.

As a teenager, I escaped my upbringing for a while. I threw away the clunky shoes, took up a sport, lost weight, and began to attract some welcome male attention. My foot problem inspired me to study podiatry, and a few short years later I had a thriving professional practice, a husband, two children, and absolutely no time to myself.

I regressed to my old habits. I no longer did anything more strenuous than walking to the refrigerator, and I steadily and undramatically gained weight. At 29, I weighed a whopping 180 pounds, a heavy load for a 5-foot-4 frame. It was weight I could no longer hide, even with the most clever clothing. Three months after the birth of my second child, people thought I was still pregnant. That's when I knew I had to do *something*.

Searching for that something was a long journey. My experience reads like a social history of exercise and diet in the 1970s and '80s. I bought every tape Jane Fonda ever made, but her program was such a grinding chore that I couldn't make myself do the exercises. My bedroom decor includes a $3,000 computerized indoor bicycle and an $800 cross-country skiing machine, both very handy to drape clothes on.

I signed up for aerobic dance at a swanky health club, hoping that the large financial investment would increase my motivation. How I cringed from all those mirrors reflecting my heavy body squeezed into a leotard. And I felt like a klutz. I didn't learn the routines easily, and the indifference of the instructors and the thinness and grace of the other students soon made me dread going. A try at ballet class ended the same way. "Never too late to start," chirped the ads, but the class was full of lithe-limbed, long-necked ladies *resuming* ballet.

Jogging, roller skating, and bike riding also bit the dust. The jogging was torture on my knees, feet, and back. After six miserable weeks, I finally came to the conclusion that jogging is for those genetically endowed with tall bodies, long limbs, good joint alignment, and legs of even length. And bicycling is for those handy with tools; my bike was always in the shop with a flat tire or malfunctioning gearshift.

After a year of dauntless experimenting with various kinds of exercises, the gods finally took pity on me. It was a lovely day in June and I was in a big hurry to get home from my office. I tried to hail a cab for several frustrating minutes and finally decided that I'd walk—high heels, briefcase, shopping bag, and all. Since I had someone waiting at home, I walked at quite a fast pace—less than a minute a block.

As I walked, I noticed that my mind was cleansed of all the minor annoyances of the day. I watched the passing faces on the street with interest, and familiar places took on a new freshness. When I reached my home, I realized, to my surprise, that I felt terrific. My breathing was a bit faster and deeper than normal, but I wasn't uncomfortable. My skin looked bright from the rushing air. Although I'd just worked for nine hours, I felt more refreshed and energetic than when I'd woken up in the morning.

This incident occurred in 1984, when walking was not generally considered a form of exercise. But as a doctor, I knew that the goal of exercise was increased heart rate and muscle use, and that there was no reason these could not be achieved by brisk walking. Then and there I decided to drop all guilt feelings about the expensive clotheshorses in the bedroom and the lapsed health-club member-ships. I was going to walk—every day—and I was going to do it because I liked it, because doing so felt comfortable, because it was "me."

This promise to myself turned out to be surprisingly easy to keep. For the past six years, I have, in fact, walked almost every day. Most of the time I walk around the track in New York's Central Park, ignoring the disdain of joggers who try to push me out of the way. But sometimes, if I can't make the park, I take my hour on the city's streets, or the roads near our country home.

After six months of walking, I gained so much confidence and control over my life that I was at last really ready to tackle my weight problem. By itself, walking took off some of the pounds—but the process was very slow. I had tried even more diets than exercise programs (see Part 4, "The Walker's Diet," for details), but this time I had the confidence to create my own diet, based on the foods I like to eat, my schedule, and my basic knowledge of good nutrition. In a year and a half, I lost 60 pounds.

Can walking work for you as it did for me? I believe walking is the exercise answer for many types of people:

- the nonathletic
- the over-35 crowd
- those with medical problems
- those who don't like to exercise
- those with very busy, unpredictable schedules

Walking has become one of the most reliably pleasurable parts of the day. Although I was a woman who had everything—a successful career, a happy marriage, children, friends—I now have something even more: I have part of the day reserved for myself. I control it. I'm indisputably in charge. And I don't have to depend on anyone else's time or mood to use it.

How This Program Is Different

This book begins with the pleasure principle: the simple premise that it's easier to get yourself to do something you like than something you don't like. Walking is the most "likable" exercise for nonathletic people. It's pleasantly private. When you use the Walk It Off! system, passersby won't even know you're exercising, and you might forget it yourself. And walking can be combined with other enjoyable activities—window shopping, cloud gazing, socializing.

The Walk It Off! system is also self-adjusting. You can begin with a very gentle program that's ideal for people trying to ease themselves into an exercise habit, and for people with injuries or medical problems. It can also be turned into a highly strenuous workout for the person who is ready for more.

But is walking "real" exercise? Indeed it is, and more and more doctors are finding that it is also the safest, most agreeable, and most accessible exercise they can recommend to their patients. And although there's no one "right" way to walk, there are a number of tricks of the trade that experienced walkers have discovered.

The Walk It Off! technique is designed to be failure-proof, even for those who, like me, have managed to flunk every other exercise program on the market. What makes it failure-proof is that it's built on your own assessment of what you enjoy doing, your age, your health condition, your life-style, and your personal and social environment.

There are no "right" answers on the simple tests and mental exercises included throughout this book. They're designed to make you think about your daily life in a new way and to find out how active you really are at home and on the job, what types of situations are most likely to make you feel good, and how you can make walking a part of your personal daily schedule.

Part 1, "Getting Started," is intended to begin this process of introducing walking into your life. The walking program itself—described in Chapter 3, "The Happy Walker"—is devised to help you increase your activity level, gradually and painlessly. The program teaches you to warm up both mind and muscles and start walking at a comfortable level that will make you feel good as well as fit.

But as I know from long experience, starting an exercise program is not the same as sticking to it. Too little attention has been paid to the art of building a new habit—which, by definition, is something that's easier to keep than to break. In Part 2, "Building a Walking Habit," I show you how to acquire such a habit using solid health information, psychological tips, and self-rewards.

Part 3, "On the Road," deals with the practical aspects of life on the hoof. What should you do if it rains? If a dog chases you? If you develop a blister? If you get bored with the whole routine?

The Walk It Off! weight-loss plan is discussed in Part 4, "The Walker's Diet." The eating plan is unlike any you're likely to have met before. Diet suggestions not only incorporate the latest information about how to lose weight permanently, but also emphasize food selections that are known to give other health benefits, such as reducing the risk of heart disease and osteoporosis.

Part 5, "The Healthy Walker," explains what to do about foot problems and includes a chapter of answers to a variety of questions about walking and health, some of concern to all walkers, others of concern to older walkers and those with special limitations or disabilities.

Part 6, "Advanced Walking," is for the convinced walker—the person with a serious walking habit—the person you will be just ninety days after you begin the Walk It Off! program. The chapters in this part show how your powerful new habit can become a great source of recreation and social life. How it can help you cope with any medical problems or limitations as you age. And, perhaps most important, how it can make you feel happier and more positive about yourself.

Walk It Off! is an invitation to take a fresh and positive look at your life, to discover what really makes you happy, and to use that self-knowledge to work out a walking routine that just might become the most pleasurable part of your day.

PART

1

GETTING STARTED

If this book were merely about "how to walk," I could cover the ground in a few pages, like the pamphlets given out by walking-shoe companies. For walking is, indeed, among the simplest sports. You don't need to learn many new skills or acquire difficult technical knowledge.

But making health walking a regular part of your daily routine takes some doing. For those of us who are not natural exercisers, finding time, energy, and motivation to walk requires a major life change. We may wish we could just snap our fingers and "decide" to do it. But, in fact, it takes a steady build-up of mental, emotional, and physical energy to work into a new habit. To start, you'll need to have a bit of patience with yourself. It will take some thought to analyze your own daily habits and figure out how walking can fit into your personal routine.

This first section will help you do just that. It will also help you learn—by doing—how a modest 20-minute walk can have a major enhancing effect on your health, your energy level, and your mood.

> *Walking 20 minutes* at least four or five times a week is how the President's Council of Fitness and Sports recommends you begin. The eventual goal is walking 3 miles in 45 minutes comfortably, but there is no hurry in getting there.

1

Walking and You

When I started walking, in 1984, there were mostly joggers in the park. I seldom saw another walker. I started in the early winter, which was really ideal for someone who weighed 178 pounds. I could hide in my winter clothing and feel less self-conscious as those long-legged, energetic joggers passed me by around the track in New York's Central Park.

I began to walk in the morning, for much the same reason. Few people were out, especially as it got colder, and I didn't feel I was on display. Of course, my husband thought I was nuts and told me many times that I'd never keep it up. Hadn't he seen the bills for the exercise machines and tennis outfits that lay abandoned in the bedroom? "Where are you going so early?" he'd ask me those first few weeks. "It's freezing out. You'll never lose weight walking."

What kept me going? Certainly I'd started, and flunked, enough other exercise programs to fill a college catalog. But this wasn't an aerobic dance class with relentless mirror images of myself out of step with the other bouncing beauties to bring me down. And this wasn't running after missed balls on the tennis court, working up an unpleasant sweat. (*Real* athletes will tell you it makes them feel great to work up a good sweat; but the rest of us just feel—well, clammy and unattractive.)

Walking *felt good* from the very first time out, and each time after that! I saw and felt improvements in my mood, breathing, and muscle tone almost immediately. And instead of feeling like a dance failure or a tennis klutz, I focused on the clouds, the tree-tops, the hopping sparrows, the playful squirrels—*not* on myself.

The first sign that I was actually *doing something* for my body was that my legs began to itch. That meant I was increasing the circulation and flow of blood through my body. I knew it was a good sign, and after I came back from my morning walk I massaged my legs with a cream.

Running is hard on the joints because the impact of each step forces the body to absorb a shock that's three or four times your body weight. When you walk, the impact of each step is only 1 to 1.5 times your weight.

After just a week I noticed that I had less swelling in my feet and my hands. I hadn't lost much weight, but I did feel slimmer . . . and prettier! It was easier to look in the mirror. There was less puffiness under my eyes. I looked wide-awake. My skin had a pinker tone and I found I needed less makeup to face the world.

Walking seemed to have a tonic effect on my appetite, too. I didn't crave a danish in the morning for a sugar rush to get me going. I needed less coffee. In fact, I went out for my walk at 7:00 a.m. without drinking anything so I wouldn't have to go to the bathroom. When I came home, I found myself craving juice or a piece of fruit, not coffee.

In looking back, I think there were several reasons why I was able to get into the walking habit after I'd failed so many times. First of all, walking emphasized my strengths, not my weaknesses.

Second, it was self-reinforcing: every time I did it, I wanted to do it again. I felt good as I walked, and even better for the rest of the day, when I glowed with energy and a sense of well-being.

(Later on, we'll talk about creating rewards for yourself each time you get out and walk, as a way of building a habit. But though this is a nice frill, it's not essential, for walking in itself is a reward, not a punishment.) And, probably most important, walking is *easy* to fit in to my rather nutty schedule. When I'm on the road, lecturing at health spas or corporate conventions, I may not be able to find a gym, or a class, or a swimming pool. But there's always a country road, a sidewalk, or a park available, and all I have to do is remember to pack some comfortable clothes and shoes.

Okay, that's enough about *me*. What about you? If at this point what you're really dying to do is put on your sneakers and go out for a walk, go for it. You can always read the rest of the book when you get back.

But at some point, now or later, you'll need to give a little thought to your own past experiences with exercise, your beliefs about walking, and the other obligations in your life (work, family, hobbies). I don't intend to recommend years of psychoanalysis to accomplish this. Instead, all you need is a pencil and a few minutes to answer the quick quizzes that follow.

"We are underexercised as a nation. We look instead of play. We ride instead of walk. Our existence deprives us of the minimum of physical activity essential for healthy living."—JOHN F. KENNEDY

There are no right or wrong answers to these tests. They're designed to help you access your own experiences and attitudes and help you plan your way around any obstacles that may exist to your developing a walking habit.

After the quizzes, I suggest various ways you can use your answers to plan a walking program that suits yourself. But I hope you'll also find that the process of answering these questions helps you gain some insight into yourself.

A: Your Exercise Experience

1. Which of these exercises have you tried?

_____ jogging
_____ competitive running
_____ jumping rope
_____ home video exercise program
_____ daily walking
_____ race walking
_____ aerobic dance
_____ exercise machines (bikes, rowers, Nautilus, etc.)
_____ court sports (tennis, racquetball, basketball, etc.)
_____ swimming
_____ dance (ballet, tap, etc.)
_____ free weight lifting
_____ bicycling (outdoors)
_____ rowing (outdoors)
_____ skating
_____ mini-trampoline
_____ cross-country skiing
_____ mountain climbing
__12__ TOTAL NUMBER CHECKED

2. What is the longest consecutive period you've stayed with an exercise program in the past?

a. _____ 1 week
b. _____ 4 weeks
c. _____ 5–10 weeks
d. __✓__ more than 10 weeks

3. If you've dropped out of previous exercise programs, what was your reason for stopping? (Check all that apply.)

_____ boredom
_____ no time
_____ achiness or injuries
_____ too tiring

_____ wasn't good at it
_____ didn't enjoy it
_____ became inconvenient
__✓__ TOTAL NUMBER CHECKED

4. Have you ever experienced an exercise injury?

    a. _____ no   b. __✓__ yes

5. Have you ever joined a health club?

__✓__ no _____yes. If yes, how long did you attend regularly?

    a. _____ 1 week
    b. _____ 4 weeks
    c. _____ 5–10 weeks
    d. _____ more than 10 weeks

6. Have you ever enrolled in an exercise class?

    a. __✓__ no   b. _____ yes

7. Have you ever been on a weight-loss diet?

    a. __✓__ no   b. _____ yes

8. When you were a schoolchild (ages 5 to 10) were you:

    a. __✓__ highly active
    b. _____ somewhat active
    c. _____ not active

9. When you were an adolescent (ages 11 to 18) were you:

    a. __✓__ highly active
    b. _____ somewhat active
    c. _____ not active

10. What types of activities do you like to do in your spare time today?

    a. __✓__ read books, magazines, or newspapers
    b. _____ gardening
    c. __✓__ watch television
    d. _____ working around the house (fixing, cleaning, etc.)

e. _____ go to movies
f. _____ watch sporting events
g. _____ ride bicycle
h. _____ go dancing
i. _____ listen to music
j. _____ talk on the telephone
k. _____ active play with children
l. _____ cooking
m. _____ take long baths
n. _____ play tennis or other ball game
o. _____ swim
p. _____ go for drives
q. _____ shop
r. _____ eat dinner out

How to score
Question 1: 1 point for each item checked
Question 2: b - 1 point; c - 5 points; d - 10 points
Question 3: 1 point for each item checked
Question 4: b - 1 point
Question 5: b - 1 point; c - 5 points; d - 10 points
Question 6: b - 5 points
Question 7: b - 2 points
Question 8: a - 2 points; b - 1 point
Question 9: a - 2 points; b - 1 point
Question 10: 1 point for each of the following checked: b, d, g, h,
  k, l, n, o, q
TOTAL NUMBER OF POINTS _____

What Your Score Suggests
0-20: This is the kind of score I would have gotten if I had taken
this test when I was 30 years old. It reflects relatively little experience with exercise and little inclination to participate in the more
active aspects of daily living.

Even if you're currently 78 years old, there's no reason to think
of your inexperience as a drawback to starting a walking program.

In fact, you've got at least one advantage: you've probably avoided a lot of negative exercise experiences and are relatively unacquainted with exercise failure.

However, it's essential that you recognize that you are an exercise beginner. That means you should probably start at the very easiest level of the walking program and increase slowly, even ridiculously slowly. But there's no rush, is there? If you've waited all this time to start exercising there's no sense pushing too hard and ending up injured and discouraged. And remember, you've got one important thing going for you: beginner's luck!

21-44: This is the range I might have been in after five years of annoying and discouraging attempts to force myself to stick with unpleasant exercise programs. You may have spent a lot of money on health clubs, equipment, exercise videos, and even doctors to repair exercise injuries. You may even have stuck to an exercise program for six months only to lose interest and patience with it. If you dropped out, abruptly or gradually, you probably promised yourself over and over that next week, or "in the spring," you'd get going again.

As an experienced starter of exercise programs, you probably have a wealth of insight to draw on and may find it quite natural to get going on a walking routine. But exercise may also have developed some unpleasant associations for you, because you feel guilty for having spent money and then failed to carry through, or are still sore from old injuries and defeats.

Hang in there! In the pages that follow I'll show you how to drop the guilt and use what you've learned in the past to propel you into a walking future!

45-66: A score in this range means you're an old hand at all types of active living and exercise. You may now be turning to walking because injuries or a health condition have made you wary of tennis or jogging. Or you may realize that you need steady, convenient aerobic conditioning in addition to your occasional skydiving and ski trips.

As an active person, you may be wondering if walking is really worthwhile and whether it's really possible to have gain without pain. And, in fact, if you're currently in good condition, you may want to skip the beginner's program and start off on the intermediate or advanced levels.

Certainly, you're ripe for exercise. Your challenge is to make it a regular, convenient part of your life!

B: Your Exercise and Health Beliefs

1. A daily brisk walk can improve a person's mood and reduce stress.

_____ true
_____ false

2. To be really good for you, exercise should be difficult—"no pain, no gain."

_____ true
_____ false

3. People who exercise regularly see improvements in fitness with each session.

_____ true
_____ false

4. It takes great personal discipline and motivation to stick to an exercise program.

_____ true
_____ false

5. To stay fit you must constantly increase your exercise level.

_____ true
_____ false

6. Walking is not real aerobic exercise.

_____ true
_____ false

7. Exercise alone can cause weight loss.

_____ true
_____ false

8. Weight-bearing exercise helps keep bones strong and prevent osteoporosis.

_____ true
_____ false

9. The most noticeable benefits of exercise come after two or three months of regular participation.

_____ true
_____ false

10. When you feel pain during exercise, the best thing to do is keep going and work through it.

_____ true
_____ false

11. There's not much you can do to improve your health.

_____ true
_____ false

12. Ordinary walking is not good exercise; you need special techniques.

_____ true
_____ false

13. It gets harder to stick to an exercise program as time goes by.

_____ true
_____ false

14. Setting high goals from the beginning is the only way to achieve fitness.

_____ true
_____ false

15. People who have dropped exercise programs before are likely to do it again.

_____ true
_____ false

16. Walking may be okay as a beginning, but it's not enough to achieve true fitness.

_____ true
_____ false

17. Unless an exercise session leaves you sweaty and out of breath, you haven't done yourself any good.

_____ true
_____ false

18. Moderate exercise can improve a person's chances of having a longer and healthier life.

_____ true
_____ false

Answers
All the statements are false *except* 1, 7, 8, 9, and 18.
Let's look at what scientific studies have shown in the last few years.

1. A daily brisk walk can improve a person's mood and reduce stress. TRUE. There's no question that this is true. In fact, scientists have found that a daily walk elevates the mood of even severely depressed psychiatric patients. It works for the elderly, for schoolchildren, and for stressed-out working people.

2. To be really good for you, exercise should be difficult—"no pain, no gain." FALSE. The good news from scientific studies of the last few years is that pain is not only unnecessary for achieving fitness, it's not a good idea. Because the truth is, most people are not stupid enough to put up with painful exercise for very long. It's far better to do something pleasant, and stick to it, than to occasionally beat yourself up at the gym.

3. People who exercise regularly see improvements in fitness with each session. FALSE. This is the type of hyped-up expectation fostered by fitness gurus. It's nice to dream, but in fact, you probably won't have better breath and be able to walk farther and faster with each session. In fact, there will be days that you won't do as well as the week before. You may not be feeling as well, the weather may make you blue, or you may be more tired than usual. But as long as you stick to your walking program, you will see results in the long haul.

4. It takes great personal discipline and motivation to stick to an exercise program. FALSE. Not with the Walk It Off! program. It does take a moderate amount of motivation, but after you get yourself into the walking habit, the ''discipline'' is about as difficult as telling yourself you must eat dessert!

5. To stay fit you must constantly increase your exercise level. FALSE. It's not true that you can always become faster, stronger, or more flexible. Our bodies have built-in limits that are best respected. In fact, once your body is well conditioned (this takes most people about six months of walking) you may even be able to cut back on the time you spend exercising and still achieve maximum health benefits.

6. Walking is not real aerobic exercise. Walking is, indeed, excellent aerobic exercise that stimulates the heart, lungs, and muscles and increases the circulation of the blood so that it benefits every organ of the body. Your heart may not pound the way it does when you're running or dancing at a fast pace. But pink cheeks, tingly skin, and a feeling of renewed energy are the gentler signs that your walking is conditioning your heart.

7. Exercise alone can cause weight loss. TRUE. Theoretically, if you increase the amount of energy you expend and eat your usual amount of food, you should lose weight. For people who are hoping to lose, say, 5 pounds over a year, or to maintain their weight, walking alone is enough. But I don't want to kid you. If you're overweight and want to lose fairly quickly, it will also be necessary to cut back on fattening, unhealthy foods. Happily, this becomes a lot easier to do once you've established a walking habit.

8. Weight-bearing exercise helps keep bones strong and prevents osteoporosis. TRUE. During weight-bearing exercise, such as walking, the force of gravity becomes an ally. It pulls on the tissue of your bones and stimulates them to take in more calcium and maintain their density and strength. The absence of this stimulation is what causes astronauts to lose bone density in the gravity-free atmosphere of space. Regular walking and a calcium-rich diet are the best-known ways to prevent osteoporosis and the broken hips and arms and spinal distortions that limit the lives of many elderly people.

9. The most noticeable benefits of exercise come after two or three months of regular participation. TRUE. Those of you who have never stuck to an exercise program for that long have never had a chance to experience what a boost in fitness feels like. After two or three months you'll feel a new sense of power every time you climb a flight of stairs, lift a bag of groceries, or run for a bus.

10. When you feel pain during exercise, the best thing to do is keep going and work through it. FALSE. Please don't fall for this dangerous exercise myth! The fact is that a staggering three to five million sports-related injuries—some of them quite serious and even crippling—turn up every year at doctors' offices, clinics, and emergency rooms. And this statistic tells only part of the story, since it doesn't include all of the minor and major aches, pains, and pulled muscles that go unreported. The autopsy reports on running guru Jim Fixx, for example, showed he had ignored three heart attacks in the eight weeks preceding his fatal one.

If you feel any pain greater than a slight tug on your leg muscles while you're walking, stop and rest. If you don't feel better in a few minutes, call an ambulance. Pain in the chest, neck, arms, or jaw during exertion is a sign of heart problems. Even if symptoms quickly disappear, make an appointment to see a doctor.

11. There's not much you can do to improve your health. FALSE. In fact, there is, even if you're currently quite ill with a chronic disease. Walking may not help you lick the disease, but it can make you feel better on a day-to-day basis. Your improved mood will help motivate you to take your medicine, stick to your nutrition plan, and do whatever else will maximize your health.

12. Ordinary walking is not good exercise; you need special techniques. FALSE. Strolling along keeping an eye on a toddler, walking a dog that pauses and sniffs around every few yards, and window-shopping are not, of course, types of walking that condition your body. But I believe that in general, walking is better than sitting in a car. So in addition to taking your regular exercise walks, take advantage of any chance you get to walk.

13. It gets harder to stick to an exercise program as time goes by. FALSE. Even though over months and years, life (blizzards, broken ankles, sick children) will inevitably get in the way of your walking program at times, once you've gotten over the ninety-day hump and have made walking a true habit, you'll find it easier to return to after any lapses.

14. Setting high goals from the beginning is the only way to achieve fitness. FALSE. In fact, goals that are unrealistically high simply set you up for failure. Your exercise goals should be somewhat challenging, but not overwhelming.

15. People who have dropped exercise programs before are likely to do it again. FALSE. Don't let this myth defeat you. In fact, studies have shown that it often takes several tries to change an ingrained habit, such as smoking cigarettes or avoiding exercise. If you've failed in the past, you've accumulated some knowledge about what does, and doesn't, work for you. You can use that knowledge to succeed this time around.

16. Walking may be okay as a beginning, but it's not enough to achieve true fitness. FALSE. This is not true for the person with ordinary fitness goals: better health, more energy, improved mood, and aerobic conditioning. If, however, you're interested in running marathons or competing in Best Body on the Beach contests, you may want to add other exercises once you've gotten into the walking habit.

17. Unless an exercise session leaves you sweaty and out of breath, you haven't done yourself any good. FALSE. In this program, if your walk leaves you panting and dripping, you've probably done too much and should cut back a bit the next time. Remember, we're shooting for long-term health-building results, not trying to impress the neighborhood with your exertion.

18. Moderate exercise can improve a person's chances of having a longer and healthier life. TRUE. This is the most exciting news to come from scientific studies over the past few years. Moderate, painless exercise can give great health benefits. One landmark study that has been following the health of 17,000 Harvard alumni for up to forty years offers proof of the benefits of moderate exercise. The study found that alumni who burned as little as 500 calories a week in exercise had death rates 15 to 20 percent lower than those who were almost completely sedentary. An hour to 90 minutes of walking a week is about all it takes for a 150-pound man to burn those 500 calories.

I hope this chapter has helped you gain some confidence in your ability to start a walking program right now, no matter how out of shape you are or how many times you flunked gym in the past. I also hope it has helped you realize that it's not your fault if you've fallen for exercise myths in the past. It's taken American fitness experts a good fifteen years to catch on to the idea that for most people moderation, gradualism, and pleasure—rather than pain and heavy breathing—are the keys to sticking to an exercise program.

2

Walking Readiness

Now that you've considered your past exercise experiences and beliefs, let's focus on the here and now. Are you ready to embark on a walking program today, or do you need some time to think it over? Do you have a rough idea of how you can fit walking into your schedule? Do you have a plan for staying motivated once your beginner's enthusiasm wears off?

Six years ago, when I began to walk, I did it on a "one day at a time" basis, hesitant, at first, to make a firm commitment to it. After my bad experiences with aerobic dance, ballet, and indoor and outdoor bikes, I was plagued by doubts. What if I spent $50 on a snazzy pair of walking shoes one day and never put them on again? What if walking turned out to be just another broken promise to myself?

In the midst of this vacillation, my eye fell on a school paper that my daughter had brought home from kindergarten. It was labeled "Reading Readiness" and had exercises in identifying shapes designed to prepare children to recognize the letters of the alphabet.

It occurred to me that before I made a commitment to

walking at least 20 minutes a day four times a week for the rest of my life, I might need some "walking readiness" to prepare me for this new activity. After all, adding an exercise habit would be a major change in my life. Perhaps it was worth at least as much forethought as planning a party or choosing furniture.

In the past, I'd always chosen an exercise program on impulse. A friend mentioned she had lost 15 pounds doing aerobic dance and off I went to her instructor. On another occasion, a shiny brochure for an indoor skiing machine, complete with ordering form, arrived in the mail. Then a ballet studio opened just two blocks from my house and I signed up the first time I passed it. Each time, I just plunked down my money and hoped for the best.

> "My mind rebels against working out—walking helps use the body evenly. I've always taken walks between rehearsals and performances of plays I've acted in. The stage managers have always been nervous that I wouldn't get back in time for my performances. But to my credit, I've only gotten lost once—in Lincoln Park in Chicago."—HELEN HAYES, actress

But I really didn't have the stomach for another exercise failure. I wanted to succeed for the long haul, even if it took a little longer to get started. So, after some thought, I decided on a three-pronged approach to get myself ready to walk:

First, I would test myself physically, to get at least a ballpark estimate of what kind of shape I was in.

Second, I would look into the logistics of walking. Where would I do it? What time of day? What would I wear? What if it was raining? What if my feet hurt?

And third, since I could see that my self-doubts were holding me back, I knew I needed a kind of mental readiness program, a willingness to believe that I could achieve my goals.

What follows is a slightly more polished version of the walking readiness evaluation I put myself through. It involves taking a kind of personal inventory of your current fitness level, life-style, and goals. I think you'll find that these checklists and mental exercises will give you some insight into the best way to set yourself up for success in walking.

Physical Inventory

The first things to consider are your overall health and your accustomed activity level.

A. How's your health?

1. Are you currently in poor health?

_____ yes _____ no

2. Are you taking any medications?

_____ yes _____ no

3. Do you have remnants of exercise injury?

_____ yes _____ no

If you answered no to all of the questions in section A, proceed to section B. If you answered yes to any of these questions, speak to your physician before starting a walking program. Although this advice is given in every health and fitness book on the market, it's very often ignored. You may be thinking, "My health problems are minor and won't be affected by walking." Or "The medication I'm taking has absolutely no effect on exercise." Or "Walking will be the best thing for my exercise injury." And you may well be right. But I hope that you'll call your physician, anyway. He or she may have some important advice about how you should modify your walking program to fit your own special needs. And if these suggestions prevent problems down the road, you'll be setting yourself up for successful walking.

B. Have you exercised lately?

1. When was the last time you did any type of formal exercise?

    a. _____ within the last week
    b. _____ within the last month
    c. _____ more than a month ago

2. How long has it been since you exercised regularly?

    a. _____ within the last week
    b. _____ within the last month
    c. _____ more than a month ago

3. What is the longest you've ever stuck to a regular exercise program?

    a. _____ more than a year
    b. _____ more than a month
    c. _____ less than a month

If you answered *a* to all of the above questions, you can give yourself a tentative A for fitness. You're probably ready for a challenging program and should consider yourself a candidate for the intermediate or advanced walking program described in Chapter 3. However, if you answered *b* or *c* to any of the questions, you may be better off starting with the beginner's program. If you find it too easy, you can always step up. But if it's just a little easy, stick with that level. Going slow and taking it easy can actually do more to help you develop a walking habit than biting off more than you can chew.

C. Do you have an active or sedentary life-style?

1. Give yourself 1 point for each half hour a week that you do the following activities:

    _____ active play with children
    _____ vacuuming
    _____ grocery shopping

_____ mowing lawn or other yard work
_____ walking ten blocks or more
_____ social or rock dancing
_____ cleaning kitchen
_____ climbing five flights of stairs
_____ physical labor at work (lifting, etc.)
_____ house repairs
_____ TOTAL NUMBER OF POINTS

2. Approximately how many hours a week do you spend sitting (behind a desk, at the wheel of a car, in front of TV, etc.)?

a. _____ 10–29 hours a week
b. _____ 30–49 hours a week
c. _____ 50–69 hours a week

If your total number of points from question 1 is less than 30—that is, if you spend less than fifteen hours a week at the activities—and your sitting time in question 2 is over 30 hours, you have what is known as a sedentary life-style. In practical terms, that means two things. First, as a health measure, regular walking is particularly important, since you spend so much of your life sitting down. Second, you may be more out of shape than you realize and should probably start the Walk It Off! program on the beginner or intermediate level.

If you spend over 30 hours a week in active, physical work or play, and less than 30 sitting down, you have at least a moderately active life-style. This may make it easier for you to start a walking program on a higher level. However, it may also make you physically tired at times and encourage the excuse "I walk all day," to avoid regular exercise. Pay special attention to finding a time to walk that will help boost your energy level.

3. How many flights of stairs can you climb without getting out of breath?

_____ flight(s)

To answer this question, you'll need more than a pencil. If you have a flight or two of stairs in your home, climb up and down them at near your maximum speed and count how many stairs you cover before your breathing gets heavy. If you live or work in a multistory building, you can take this inventory there. Otherwise, a shopping mall or a multistory department store is a good place to try it.

If you're winded and breathing hard after just 2 flights of stairs, start at the Beginner's Level. If you can do 5 or 6 flights without feeling very tired, you're probably ready for the advanced program.

Logistical Inventory

Where will you walk? What will you wear? When will you walk?

In later chapters we'll go into these questions in greater detail. But for now all you need to decide is where and when your very first few walks will occur, and what you'll wear.

To answer these questions, you need to get out of your chair and explore your neighborhood and your closet.

Where Will You Walk?

It might sound like a cop-out, but if you have a car, it's not a bad idea to go for a drive and set the mileage counter to get an idea of the distances of places you'd be likely to walk. How far is it to the bank? The train station? The nearest park with a track? The nearest indoor shopping mall? Make a few notes about any walks that look interesting and convenient.

Then do the same thing at work. Is there a park nearby, or a school with a track? If you work in a city, search out a landmark that's about twenty blocks from your workplace that you could walk to and back during lunchtime. Or consider how you might create a walk to and from work by, say, getting off the train or bus a bit before your usual stop.

If you're not sure where there's a track or a park near your home or office, start asking people. Don't limit yourself to those you know. The runner in sweat shorts jogging in place while waiting for the light to change or the policeman or postman doing his rounds is likely to know.

The goal of this exercise is to map out at least two different walks of about 2 miles each that you'd like to take in the next week or so. Then when the day comes to start your walking program you'll be ready with a route.

What Will You Wear?

It's not yet time to go to the store and buy the snappiest jogging suit or walking shoes you can find. Instead, dig into your drawers and your closet. Try to find what I like to call "comfort clothes." This might be an old stretched-out pair of pants and a large sweatshirt, a favorite sweater that makes you feel like you're being cuddled, or that miraculous pair of jeans that both fit right and feel wonderful. Consider, too, what underwear you'll put on. Many a walker has endured an uncomfortable, rather than joyful, walk because of tight-fitting underpants that rode up.

If you have a decent pair of sneakers or even very comfortable flat shoes, those are sufficient for your walking-readiness exercise. Choose your socks carefully, though, and be sure they're not too thick or too thin for the shoe you've chosen.

After you've chosen an outfit, try it on! Jump up and down a bit in front of the mirror and walk in place. Do the comfort clothes cut, bind, ride up, or otherwise annoy you? If so, try to find a substitute. The goal is to find clothes that make you free and let you move.

Once you've chosen your "comfort" outfit, see if you can find another set of clothes, almost as comfortable, that make you *look* good. It may be just adding a colorful scarf, a dashing cap, or that blue sweater that everyone says brings out the color of your eyes.

Women might consider a flowing skirt, instead of pants, for this second outfit.

I like to wear my "comfort" outfit—an oversized navy sweatshirt and gray cloth jogging pants—on the days that I'm feeling sluggish and withdrawn. Wearing oversized clothes in muted or dark colors helps me blend into the mainstream of pedestrian traffic. Comfort clothes are for the day I don't want to be noticed or call attention to myself. If I see an old boyfriend in the street, I can just keep walking and he'll probably never notice me.

On sunny, cheery days, however, I choose my second outfit—a slim-fitting rose-colored jogging suit with white stripes down the side. I might put on a little makeup before I go out to walk and pin my hair up with a ribbon. This outfit is for days when I feel I want to connect with life, celebrate, make a positive statement, and let the world know I'm there. On days like this if I see an old boyfriend I'll want to stop and chat.

Once you've chosen walking clothes to express your own withdrawn and outgoing moods, find a special spot in a drawer or closet to put them. That way when you're ready to start the program, your "comfort" and "looking good" clothes will be ready and waiting.

When Will You Walk?

It's too soon to come up with a "lifetime" answer to this question—e.g., I will *always* walk 30 minutes before breakfast. As you get into the Walk It Off! program you'll experiment with several times of day to find those that fit most easily into your schedule.

All you need to do at this point is decide when you're going to take your first two walks. If you're starting this program in cold weather, try to pick a time during the warmer part of the day. If it's the heat of summer, early morning or sundown is a better choice.

If you're a very busy person, the challenge is to find a time to "sneak in" a walk. Dog owners often think of themselves as walkers because they take the dog out a few times a day. But let's face it, the dog is the leader on most of these walks and the owner stops obediently whenever the animal wants to sniff, scratch, or talk to another dog. This kind of stop-and-go walking does not substitute for 20 to 60 minutes of brisk, steady fitness walking. The same is true of walking with a toddler in a stroller or a small child—it's stop-and-go and at a pace a lot slower than your maximum. After all, how can you give the child "quality time" if you're focused on your walking pace? So it's important to schedule your walk at a time you can leave the dog and the children at home.

Go over your plans for the next days in your mind and try to find an opening. For example, a woman I know is the mother of a toddler who had finally gotten used to being on his own in nursery school for two hours a day. The mother usually tried to jam a dozen errands into those two hours, but during her walking-readiness exercise she used that time, instead, to get started on the program.

Logistical Summary

When you've completed these exercises, write down your conclusions in the space below.

Where I'll walk:

Day 1 route:
          approximate mileage:
Day 2 route:
          approximate mileage:

What I'll wear:

top
pants or skirt
underwear
socks
shoes
outerwear

When I'll walk:

Day 1:
Day 2:

Mental Inventory

No two readers of this book are in exactly the same frame of mind when they start the Walk It Off! program. Maybe you've just stopped smoking and need to exercise off your anxiety. Or you may have learned that osteoporosis runs in your family and may be determined to do whatever you can to prevent being bent over as you get older. Or perhaps you've just separated from your spouse and desperately need something to make you feel good about yourself.

Now is the time to consider which walking goals are more important to you right now. Later I'll show you how you can use your own customized goals to keep yourself motivated. For now, just identify these goals.

Walking Wish List

1. Check all of the goals you hope to achieve from walking:

 _____ increase my strength
 _____ improve my endurance
 _____ improve my breath
 _____ condition my heart
 _____ condition my muscles
 _____ improve my posture
 _____ help prevent disease
 _____ help me feel and stay young
 _____ improve my sex drive
 _____ enjoy nature
 _____ explore city or suburban neighborhood

_____ tone my body to look thinner

_____ improve body contours (flatten stomach, thin thighs, etc.)

_____ reach peak physical condition

_____ do the minimum exercise necessary for good health

_____ improve my mood

_____ prepare for hiking

_____ give myself a break

_____ lose weight

_____ maintain my weight

_____ cope with difficult work situation

_____ cope with personal difficulties

_____ reduce stress

_____ take some time for myself

_____ feel stronger

_____ feel more energetic

_____ make friends

_____ have time alone

2. Now select the goals that are _most_ important to you at the moment, the ones that really motivated you to buy this book. You can put a star next to those in the list above. If you put a star next to more than three goals, go back to your list again and choose the three of those that are most important right now.

Reason #1 _____

Reason #2 _____

Reason #3 _____

Walking Readiness in Action

If you've considered how fit you are at the moment, where and when you'll begin to walk and what you'll wear, and why you're embarking on this program, you've already achieved walking readiness.

This is a much bigger step than it may seem. You've already

begun to make a commitment. You've taken the time to think through how you'll manage the program.

To show you just how big a step it is, I'd like to tell you about two people I know for whom the small step of getting themselves ready to walk was the beginning of major, positive changes in their lives.

Take This Job and Shove It

When Robert J. signed up for my Walk It Off! program at his workplace, he was at a low ebb in his life. Although the 43-year-old circulation manager had long been meaning to do something about exercise and was concerned with his health, his immediate motivations were more specific. His old boss and mentor had recently been transferred to another department, and Robert was not getting along with his new boss.

So in his walking-readiness inventory Robert decided his most important goals were to:

- cope with his difficult work situation
- reduce stress
- feel stronger

He walked with my Walk It Off! group for just two sessions, learning the warm-ups and the stride, and then decided that spending that time with his coworkers was not helping him reduce stress. So after work one day he explored the neighborhood near his plant and discovered a small, pleasant park.

The next week Robert J. was so angry at his boss that he tore out of the office as soon as a particularly annoying business meeting ended. His stomach was all in knots and he didn't want to eat, so he headed for the park and "paced around it like a madman, stomping out my anger."

He found that a good, fast-paced 15-to-20-minute walk did indeed fulfill his goals. He spent the first few minutes rerunning the frustrations of the morning, complete with mutterings of "I can't believe my boss is so stupid" and "I should have told him exactly what I think." This allowed him to get in touch with the emotions he had to suppress during working hours and also to clear his mind so he could *think* clearly and calmly about how to handle the situation. He found the walk much more relaxing than a two-martini lunch or gulping down a sandwich at his desk while shuffling through phone messages.

Robert began to take a lunchtime walk every day when the weather was at least passably good. It helped him separate himself physically and mentally from his job and to evaluate his situation objectively. On particularly rough days, he tried to take another short walk before he went home so that he didn't bring his irritations home to his family.

Walking proved to be an excellent form of career therapy for Robert. He eventually realized that he was never going to enjoy working with his new boss, and he applied for, and eventually got, a transfer to another department. He still takes noontime walks, but these days does a whole lot less "stomping." And his early goals have changed from stress reduction and coping to improving his health and fitness.

Too Many Hours in the Day

Jenny L., 62, was in for her fourth doctor's appointment in several months. She'd been having difficulty sleeping and often found herself short of breath from the slightest exertion. Her physician had given her a complete physical and round of laboratory tests. She told Jenny that all the test results were normal, and then began to inquire gently into how Jenny was spending her time.

"Oh, I don't do much anymore," was Jenny's reply. Her husband had died a year before and her children were grown and living in distant cities. Jenny no longer enjoyed her work as a secretary, and so when her corporation offered a sizable financial bonus to employees who took early retirement, she took them up on their offer.

> *Simply taking time off* from the strains of everyday life is one of the most important benefits of walking. It helps you clarify and focus your thinking and increases feelings of contentment.

Now, at 62, Jenny had neither spouse, children, nor job to schedule her life around. After a few weeks of luxuriating in sleeping late and watching daytime television for the first time in her life, Jenny began to panic. Far from enjoying her freedom, she found she hated waking up each day with nothing in particular to do. And while she wasn't exactly sick, she never felt well enough to get involved in new activities.

Jenny's doctor referred her to me to get her started on a walking program. Jenny had a lot of difficulty deciding on her walking-readiness goals. It took days for her to bring herself to choose an outfit to wear and a time of day to leave the house. But choose she did, at last. Her mental goals were to:

- improve her breath
- get out of the house
- improve her mood

And, indeed, after a long preparatory period, Jenny got started. Instead of turning on the television in the morning, or even *thinking* about how she felt, she got right into a jogging suit and was out the door after drinking a glass of orange juice. Jenny slept so poorly that often she was wide awake at dawn and just waiting for it to get light enough for her walk.

In just a week's time, the walking began to have a profound effect on Jenny's life. The new routine helped diminish her anxiety, which the doctor thought was the source of her breathing difficulties and insomnia. Jenny began to really notice what was going on in her neighborhood and found herself recognizing and greeting the other morning regulars who were out sweeping the sidewalk in front of their stores. The walk got her "juices flowing" so that when she returned home she was full of ideas about how she might spend the rest of the day. She began by completing projects around the house—repapering the kitchen shelves and redecorating a bathroom. By the fourth week of walking, she felt well enough to drop in at the volunteer service agency she had been meaning to sign up with and also to pick up some booklets about community center activities in her neighborhood.

When Jenny returned for her next scheduled doctor's appointment, after a month of walking, she could report that she was sleeping a lot better and almost never had that constricted, short-of-breath feeling in her chest. Instead of seeing her life as a yawning gap of time to fill, she now relishes the adventure of planning her own days. For Jenny, the morning walk was the first step in liberating her spirit from grief at the loss of her husband and job.

3

The Happy Walker

Okay. It's time to declare yourself "ready." You have an idea where you're going to take those first few walks, what you're going to wear, and what your goals are—what's in it for you.

The rest is a matter of doing it: taking action. Get into one of your walking outfits; do the simple exercises in the 3-minute warm-up and 2-minute psych-up sessions that follow; and seize the reward you deserve: a brisk, lively, determined, happy half hour outdoors.

The 3-Minute Stretch

Why stretch? For one thing, if you do it right (gently, slowly, kindly, to music if you like) it feels good! Anyone who's ever watched a cat waking from a nap has observed the kind of sensual pleasure that stretching can bring.

Stretching also helps make walking a pleasant, pain-free

experience. When we walk we're working our muscles against the force of gravity. Muscles work by tightening, contracting, getting shorter. Stretching lengthens and loosens the muscles and gets them ready to work.

Stretching is especially important if you haven't exercised in quite a while, because it can save you aches and pains later on. And it's also important for energetic, advanced walkers to help avoid pain, shin splints, ligament injuries, and arthritis.

But like anything else, stretching can be overdone. Remember: always stretch with a slow, smooth, relaxed movement. Jerking, bouncing, bobbing, or pulling on your muscles can do more harm than good! And don't hold your breath. Slow, steady breathing will help your muscles relax.

I like to stretch at the front door just before I go out. This stretching routine takes only 3 minutes, so it can also be done on the ride down in the elevator or on the street.

| Side Stretch |

Goal: to stretch trunk
Repetitions: 5 times each side, hold for count of 3
   1. Stand with feet about 12 inches apart.
   2. Place left hand on your waist.
   3. Raise right arm over your head.
   4. Pull stomach muscles in and down.
   5. Bend trunk slowly to the left to the count of 3.
   6. Hold the stretch for a count of 3.
   7. Return to upright position to count of 3.

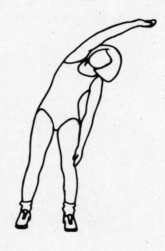

Arm Swing

Goal: to warm upper body
Repetitions: 5 times to each side
1. Stand with feet about 12 inches apart.
2. Pull stomach muscles in and down.
3. Swing arms to the right, lifting left foot onto toe.
4. Swing arms to the left, lifting right foot onto toe.

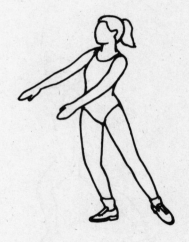

Calf Stretch

Goal: to stretch heel cord and prevent injuries
Repetitions: 1 time to each side, hold for count of 10
1. Stand with left foot in front, with knee bent.
2. Place hands on waist.
3. Keeping right leg straight, lean forward over bent knee. Keep body low and both feet on the ground.
4. Hold stretch for count of 10 (you should feel tugging in calf of right leg).

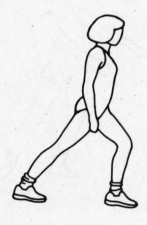

Leg Stretch (A)

Goal: to relax hamstring muscles
Repetitions: 1 time to each side; hold for count of 10
1. Put right heel on chair, table, or fence no higher than waist level.
2. With both knees straight, lean forward, try to touch right toe.
3. Hold stretch for count of 10.

Note: If this exercise is too difficult for you, substitute Leg Stretch B.

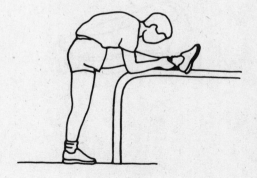

Leg Stretch (B)

Goal: to relax hamstring muscles
Repetitions: 1 time to each side, hold for count of 3
1. Sit on floor with legs straight out in front.
2. Point toes up, with heels close together.
3. With back straight, reach toward toes as far as feels comfortable.
4. Hold for count of 3.

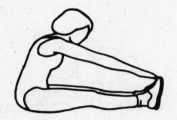

The Stork

Goal: to stretch quadriceps (the large thigh muscle)
Repetitions: 1 time each side, hold for count of 20

1. Use a chair or wall for balance if necessary.
2. Stand on left foot; bend right foot back at the knee and grasp the toe.
3. Pull right foot up until you feel a tug.
4. Hold for count of 20.

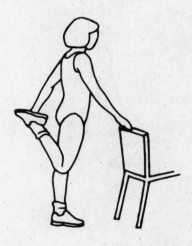

Toe Tapping

Goal: to stretch anterior muscle, up front of leg
Repetitions: 10 times for each foot
1. With weight on left foot, point right toe forward.
2. Tap 2 times forward.
3. Point right toe to side and tap 2 times.

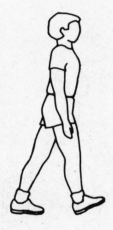

The 2-Minute Psych-up

Now that you've stretched your limbs, it's time to psyche yourself into readiness for your walk. If you can remember the word HAPPY, you'll have no trouble memorizing this exercise, which should be repeated every 5 minutes or so during your walk.

Psych-up

Goal: to improve walking posture and self-image

Repetitions: 4. Stand in front of a mirror (preferably a full-length one) and smile at yourself. Then check yourself from head to foot:

1. **Head erect, stretch up your neck.** Look yourself in the eye, stand tall, and smile. Imagine you have a crown on your head and must stretch your neck to hold it up.
2. **Arms: swing in a steady rhythm.** Bend arms at elbow and swing alternately forward.
3. **Press your shoulders down.** We tend to hunch up as we walk. Squeeze your shoulders down and back.
4. **Press in on the abdomen and breathe deeply.** Squeeze your stomach muscles in and flatten the gut. Breathe in and out to make sure you're not holding your breath.
5. **Y-step in place.** With each step, roll from outer portion of heel onto the ball of the foot with toes splaying.

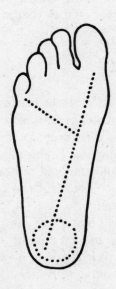

Your First Walks

Now it's time simply to leave the house and start your walk. Don't worry too much about your stride or how fast you're going during your first few walking days. Just get out there and do it, and when you get home remember to record your experience in your log.

After you've had a few days of experience in stretching, psyching up, and taking some walks, it's time to choose a regular, consistent walking program. This consists of the following steps:

- Make a commitment to walk at least four times a week and decide when during the day it's easiest for you to do it.
- Choose a walking level (beginner, intermediate, or advanced) and follow the table on page 56 to gradually increasing your time and distance.
- Read the section later in this chapter headed "How to Walk" and incorporate its advice into your steps each day.

Your Walking Level

In Chapter 2 you began to evaluate whether you should start out on the beginner, intermediate, or advanced walking level. If you're over 45, have done little or no exercise for more than a year, get out of breath from climbing two flights of stairs, or have a serious health problem, you should start out on the beginner's level. If it feels a little too easy, that's fine. If it's so easy it's boring, then go up to the intermediate level.

Those who are in fairly good shape, have an active life-style, or have been exercising on and off for the last year will probably prefer the intermediate level. If you're a very active person in excellent health, you may want to start directly on the advanced level.

Warning to the impatient and ambitious: There are no extra points in this program for skipping steps and starting out at an unrealistically advanced level. The goal is to stick to the program for the rest of your life. So it doesn't matter where you start; what matters is where you're going.

3-Mile Fitness Test

If you're still not sure which group you belong to, or if you'd simply like to get a more precise measure of how fit you are to begin with, you can take this fitness pre-test. You'll need to find a track or measure out a 3-mile stretch of level terrain for walking. Then, keeping track of the time, you simply walk the 3 miles as fast as you can without running. Write down how many minutes it took you to walk the 3 miles, then check the results against the table below to determine your walking group.

Note: Check with your doctor before taking this test if you have health problems or are over 35 and don't exercise regularly.

MEN

Age	20–29	30–39	40–49	50–59	over 60
Beginner	>42 min.	>43 min.	>45 min.	>48 min.	>52 min.
Intermediate	36–42 min.	37–43 min.	39–45 min.	41–48 min.	43–52 min.
Advanced	<36 min.	<37 min.	<39 min.	<41 min.	<43 min.

WOMEN

Age	20–29	30–39	40–49	50–59	over 60
Beginner	>43 min.	>45 min.	>48 min.	>50 min.	>55 min.
Intermediate	38–43 min.	40–45 min.	41–48 min.	44–50 min.	47–55 min.
Advanced	<38 min.	<40 min.	<41 min.	<44 min.	<47 min.

Take the Pulse Test, if You Must

If you've ever taken an aerobic dance class or been trained on a circuit of exercise machines, you have had lessons in taking your pulse. You've probably also been given a complicated formula for figuring out the maximum safe pulse rate for your age group. Is all that really necessary?

In my opinion, it is not necessary for most reasonably healthy people with a good dose of common sense. The "target heart rate" was invented for research purposes; it's a type of measurement that makes it possible to compare the physiological effects of various exercise regimens.

For most of us, there are less complicated ways to know if we're overtaxing our hearts. The Walk It Off! program is not a very strenuous one and should not result in a very rapid heart rate. So if you find it hard to breathe when you're walking, slow down. If you're walking so fast that you find it difficult to talk, slow down. Nausea, pain, dizziness, confusion, or irregular heart rhythm are warning signs that you need to stop exercising and seek medical advice.

However, many doctors do recommend pulse monitoring for patients who have had a heart problem, high blood pressure, high cholesterol level, or a family history of heart disease. That's the reason I recommend that if you have a health problem you consult your physician before starting a walking program.

For those who should take their pulse (and those who simply like to), here's a simple 10-second test:

- Take your pulse immediately after stopping exercise.
- Find your pulse with your index finger, not your thumb. The pulse is easiest to locate on the side of the neck or the wrist.
- Using a watch or clock with a second hand, count the number of heartbeats in a 10-second interval.
- Multiply that figure by 6 for beats per minute.
- Calculate your maximum safe heart rate by subtracting your

age from 220. (For example, if you're 40 years old, your maximum heart rate is 180 beats per minute.)
- Your pulse after exercising should be no more than 60 percent of your maximum heart rate, or 108 beats per minute if you're 40 years old.

If your pulse rate is below your target zone (50–60 percent of the maximum for your age) you will need to walk faster to get an aerobic effect. This may take a while, however, because you have to build up muscle strength in order to comfortably walk faster.

If your pulse rate is above your target zone, you're walking too fast! Slow your pace and try again. If your heartbeat easily vaults above the target zone, consult your doctor.

How to Walk

I know, you've been doing it since you were a baby. But the first few times you go out for an exercise walk, you may feel like a rank beginner. What do you do with your hands? How do you increase your walking speed without tripping over your own feet?

The HAPPY exercise at the beginning of this chapter is a good one to repeat as you walk; it will help draw you into the correct posture and attitude.

Start your walk at a brisk but comfortable pace to warm up your muscles. After about five minutes, increase your speed and shift from strolling to striding. Doing so involves both increasing the length of each step and increasing the number of steps you take per minute. If you're tall or have long legs, put most of your effort into increasing the length of your stride, covering more distance with each step. Shorter folks with short legs (like me) find it easier to take more steps per minute than to take longer ones. Don't fight your physiology! Instead, work with it and increase your walking speed with the method most comfortable for you.

One trick I've discovered for easy walking is to concentrate on your arms and your breathing, not your legs. If you hold your hands down straight as you walk, the blood will pool in them and they'll feel uncomfortably swollen. So keep your arms bent almost at a right angle. Keep your shoulders relaxed and hold your head high to make room for your diaphragm to expand.

The sit-up effect of strengthening the abdominal muscles and thus preventing back pain can be achieved while walking. Make sure your shoulders are erect and back and your buttocks tucked in.

Start by strolling easily and letting your arms swing forward from the shoulder blades. Your arms will naturally swing to counterbalance your feet. As your right foot swings forward, your left arm swings with it.

As you warm up, concentrate on swinging your arms more actively. If you bend your arms at the elbow, you can pump them faster. You'll find that your legs will naturally move faster and more vigorously to keep pace with your arms. You can increase the aerobic benefits of brisk walking by swinging your arms so that your hands reach shoulder level. The use of hand weights is discussed in Chapter 15. It's important to wait until you've completed the advanced-level program to add weights.

As you shift from strolling to striding, your stride lengthens and narrows. With each step, the leading leg pulls you forward as your trailing leg pushes off the ground. This alternatively stretches and relaxes the muscles in both the front and back of your legs. This leads to a firmer gait and stronger, more flexible legs.

Striding also loosens your hips, which become more flexible, and tightens the lower abdominal muscles, making for a stronger, flatter stomach. As you swing your arms, you'll reach farther with your hips. The more you stretch your hips, the more you'll improve your shape.

How Fast?

Brisk walking feels good. In fact, it's less tiring than strolling or slow walking. The continuous forward momentum of a brisk walk takes some of the weight of gravity off your feet. You get on a roll.

A simple way to find out how fast you're walking is to count how many steps you take per minute. Then you can use this simple conversion table to calculate your speed per hour, which is based on an average stride length of 30 inches.

Steps per minute	Minutes per mile	Miles per hour
70	30	2
90	24	2.5
105	29	3
120	17	3.5
140	15	4
160	13	4.5
175	12	5
190	11	5.5

Although it's certainly not necessary to count your steps each time you go out for a walk, I recommend you check your pace every few weeks to gauge your improvement. Here are some of the characteristics of walking at different speeds that can also help you recognize and increase your pace.

1 mile per hour

Arm movement: Swing arms naturally, letting gravity do the work.
Foot movement: Take slow, strolling, short stride.
Breathing: Breathe very naturally; you should be unaware of any exertion.
Calories burned: 30–40 a mile

2 miles per hour

Arm movement: Consciously swing arms at your side, with relaxed shoulders.

Foot movement: Walk naturally, but rhythmically.

Breathing: Breathe more actively, being aware of exhaling and inhaling; in through the nose, out through the mouth.

Calories burned: 40 to 60 a mile

3 miles per hour

Arm movement: Walk with arms swinging at 60-degree angle or more

Foot movement: Consciously elongate stride, take bigger steps.

Breathing: Distend your abdomen on inhaling, try to exhale completely; you should still be able to converse.

Calories burned: 60 to 80 a mile

4 miles per hour

Arm movement: Bend elbows at 90-degree angle between hip and chest; swing each arm forward not across the body

Leg movement: Take elongated and more frequent steps, as when quickly climbing a flight of stairs

Breathing: Breath quickens but does not become panting; you should still be able to converse without becoming winded.

Calories burned: 80 to 100 a mile

Another way to set a good pace as you walk is to sing. I sing to myself if there are other people around and out loud if I'm alone.

Get yourself walking at a good, comfortable, but slightly strenuous pace and then find a favorite song that has the same rhythm. For example, I warm up to the song "New York, New York," which has a loping, swinging pace. Then I step more quickly to the marching pace of George M. Cohan's patriotic favorite "Over There." And when I'm really going strong, I walk to the fast, hot, swinging step of "La Bamba."

If you like to count and have a stopwatch, you can measure your pace by counting how many steps you take per minute; 120 steps per minute is a good, brisk pace.

How Often?

The ideal way to build a walking habit is to do it every Monday through Friday, especially at the beginning. This will make it a part of your daily routine and give you exposure to various types of weather. And its very regularity will help you remember to do it.

If you succeed in walking five days during the week, you can then take Saturday and Sunday off without feeling guilty! If, on the other hand, you've skipped a day or two during the week, you can make them up on the weekend.

In the Walk It Off! program, which aims to build strength and endurance as well as regularity, Week 4 is purposely designed as an "easy" week. You're asked to walk only three days, and for the pace and distance of Week 1. This offers you a kind of reward for sticking to the program, and also lets your body relax after being pushed hard for three weeks.

The following six-week plan is designed to get you started in a regular walking program. Remember, it takes a minimum of ninety days to firm up a walking habit. After you've completed six weeks at one level, simply repeat the sixth week until you feel ready to increase the challenge. Then begin the six-week plan at the next level. Don't worry if it takes you months of walking to be able to move up; not everyone will be physically able to reach the advanced level. Those who do, and are ready to go beyond it, can see Chapter 15 for further challenges.

A Six-Week Plan

Week 1

Time:	30 minutes
Frequency:	4–5 times a week
Distance	
Beginner:	1 mile
Intermediate:	1½ miles
Advanced:	2 miles

Week 2

Time:	30 minutes
Frequency:	4–5 times a week
Distance	
Beginner:	1 mile
Intermediate:	1½ miles
Advanced:	2 miles

Week 3

Time:	40 minutes
Frequency:	4–5 times a week
Distance	
Beginner:	1¼ miles
Intermediate:	2 miles
Advanced:	2¼ miles

Week 4

Time:	30 minutes
Frequency:	4–5 times a week
Distance	
Beginner:	1 mile
Intermediate:	1.5 miles
Advanced:	2 miles

Week 5

Time:	50 minutes
Frequency:	4–5 times a week
Distance	
Beginner:	1½ miles
Intermediate:	2¼ miles
Advanced:	3 miles

Week 6

Time:	60 minutes
Frequency:	3 times a week
Distance:	
Beginner:	2 miles
Intermediate:	2½ miles
Advanced:	4 miles

After the Walk

Often the first thing I want to do when I come home after my walk is to drink a glass of water. Thirst is a positive sign of exertion, so greet it as a signal that you've done a good job. Sip the water slowly. If you gulp large amounts, your stomach will feel bloated and uncomfortable.

It's a good idea to do the 3-minute stretch again after your walk, especially if you notice any soreness or tiredness in your muscles. Stretch slowly, paying attention to how tingly your skin feels and how pleasant it is to be physically tired. While you're stretching, note your mood.

Use your Walker's Log (see the sample log pages in the back of this book) to record the date, time, and length of your walk. Use the comments section to note any effect it had on your mood.

If you've perspired a lot, you'll probably want to head for the shower next. Don't rush through it. See if you can't spare some moments to soak, or scrub, or smooth on some skin cream. You've just done something wonderful for yourself. You deserve at least a small reward!

The Happy Walker—in a Nutshell

The 3-Minute Stretch

- Side stretch: 5 times each side, hold for count of 3
- Arm swing: 5 times to each side
- Calf stretch: 1 time to each side, hold for count of 10
- Leg stretch: 1 time to each side, hold for count of 10
- The stork: 1 time to each side, count of 20
- Toe tapping: 10 times, each foot

The 2-Minute Psych-up

H.A.P.P.Y.:

- Head erect, stretch up your neck.
- Arms: swing in a steady rhythm.
- Press your shoulders down.
- Press in on the abdomen and breathe deeply.
- Y-step in place.

The Walk

- Walk a minimum of 20 minutes a day, four or five times a week.
- Gradually build up time walked to 60 minutes a session.
- Gradually increase speed and distance walked.
- Check posture by repeating HAPPY steps as you walk.
- Cool down afterward by walking slowly and stretching.

PART

2

BUILDING A WALKING HABIT

How often have you been so rushed in the morning that you didn't have time to brush your teeth? Very seldom, I bet. Habits like brushing your teeth are so automatic that unless you're running from a flaming apartment or rushing a loved one to the hospital, you always find time to do it.

The goal of the Walk It Off! program is to make a daily walk so much a part of your everyday routine that it will take little conscious effort to make time for it or remember to do it. In fact, doing it will be easier than not doing it.

The good news is that creating a new habit—or a positive addiction—is a lot easier than giving up an old habit, like smoking, overeating, or heavy drinking. That's because walking is not going to deprive you of anything. Instead, it will add something pleasurable and satisfying to your life.

How do you go about acquiring a healthy new habit? Public health researchers have found—and my own experience confirms—that motivation to change involves at least three factors: health information, self-esteem, and internal and external rewards. Strategies to bolster all of the components of motivation are included in the Walk It Off! program. The idea is to use them whenever you feel your desire to walk weakening.

> *Because it is virtually injury-free,* walking has the lowest dropout rate of any form of exercise.

I believe these strategies can work for you—no matter how many exercise programs you've dropped in the past, how overweight you are, how discouraged and disgusted with yourself you are, or how lazy you think you are. In my practice as a podiatrist and in my experience giving walking seminars as part of corporate fitness programs, I've learned that successful walkers come in all shapes, sizes, colors, and ages, from all different kinds of backgrounds, and with all sorts of personalities.

Each person begins to walk for his or her own reasons, but those who develop a true walking habit have one secret in common—the main reason that they walk is that they *like* to. Walking makes them feel more serene and confident. After a month or two, people get hooked on walking because it gives them a terrific afterglow, similar to the ''runner's high'' you may have heard about.

But before you get hooked, before you achieve that ''walker's high,'' you have to get out there and do it for a while. The next three chapters are designed to help break you in to the walking habit. Read them over whenever you find you don't feel like going out for a walk.

4

The Facts

I know, from bitter experience, that getting started is the *easy* part of any exercise program or diet. With the enthusiasm of a convert, I've rushed into dozens of self-reform programs only to find that a few months or even weeks later, my enthusiasm has been replaced by lethargy and dread.

When I began to commit myself to a daily walk, I searched for ways to keep my enthusiasm from dying. Rather to my surprise, I found that what worked was *not* empty pep talks by exercise experts. What kept me going, on days when I preferred not to stir out of my chair, was my knowledge of the facts. Recalling all that I knew about how exercise could keep me in great physical and mental health made my momentary laziness seem insignificant.

Recent scientific research into habit-building confirms my own experience. The human intellect is a powerful force, and the "cognitive" psychologists have found that reason is an excellent motivator.

This chapter is aimed at convincing you that time you spend walking each day is a good investment in your future. You probably already have at least a vague idea that exercise is *good* for you. But this chapter will show you how it can make a profound difference in our current and future lives.

Reread this chapter on the days that you have trouble making yourself tie on the sneakers and walk out the door. It will convince you to invest a few minutes, right now, in your health. Here are fifteen not-so-obvious reasons why you need to take your walk today:

1. You're tired.

You may not believe this until you've tried it when you're really exhausted, but a walk can actually wake you up and energize the rest of your day. The reason? Walking improves circulation to your arms and legs and stimulates the growth of the tiny blood vessels throughout your body. This improvement in collateral (extra) blood circulation leads to a greater efficiency of your entire cardiovascular system, which effectively combats the tired feeling. Walking also increases the amount of oxygen available to the brain, raises adrenaline levels, and speeds up the metabolic rate of your whole system. This leads to a mental alertness that lasts all day!

Walking certainly works better than eating a candy bar, according to researchers. Two hours after a sweet snack, research subjects reported feeling more tired and tense than those who had taken a brisk 12-minute walk two hours before. When you consume sugar you feel good for a short time because of increased glucose levels in your blood. But your pancreas is also aware of the circulating sugar and responds by secreting more insulin to neutralize it. After a short while, you're feeling droopy again and craving even more sugar, which is hard on your self-image, and your waistline.

So reach for your walking shoes, not the M&Ms!

2. You're in a bad mood.

Don't sit and stew—walk and stew. By increasing blood circulation to your muscles, walking reduces muscle tension and stimulates the release of endorphins, the natural pleasure chemicals produced by our bodies.

Exercise has such a dramatic effect on mood that many psychiatrists now use it to help treat even very severe depression. Here's the Walk It Off! formula for getting yourself out of a funk:

Use the first 10 minutes of your walk to totally concentrate on the things that are bothering you. Mentally tell off your boss, reprimand your kids, and count up all of your spouse's faults. After 10 minutes of focusing on your problem without interruptions or distractions, you're apt to get bored and even to see the other side of the issue. You'll start remembering some good things about your spouse. Why you like your job. How much worse the neighbor's kids are. As soon as your negative thinking shows a sign of slipping, shift the focus of attention outside yourself. Look at the clouds, or the trees, or the other people walking around the mall. By the time you've finished your minimum 20 minutes, your bad mood is likely to be only a memory.

3. You're hungry.

This is not a deprivation program, so if your stomach is grumbling, eat something before you go out for your walk. An apple, a couple of carrots, a glass of low-fat milk are good choices. They'll put you in the mood to do something more that's positive. When you come back from your walk you're likely to crave water, but you probably won't be hungry. The walk will reduce the nervous stress that leads to nervous snacking.

4. You want to keep your wits about you.

Walking has an invigorating effect on the brain cells. By increasing circulation, it increases the amount of nourishing oxygen available to the brain. Scientists have shown that people who exercise retain their memory, judgment, and hand-eye coordination better than sedentary folks. Nonscientists just call it "getting the dust out" of their brains.

5. You want to lose weight.

Even if you're eating exactly what you did when you were younger, you're probably gaining weight. The average person gains a pound a year after the age of 25. By age 45, that adds up to 20 pounds, or two or three clothing sizes larger. This means we need to exercise more, not less, as we get older.

Strolling at 3 miles an hour over level ground burns 240 calories an hour. Brisk walking at 4 miles an hour burns 360 calories, and fast walking at 5 or 6 miles an hour with determined arm swinging can burn about 500 calories an hour, equal to jogging.

6. Your feet hurt.

If you've gotten yourself a good pair of walking shoes, putting them on will be a delight for feet that have had a hard day in high heels or hard leather. Warm up well and walk slowly and gently at first, until your feet relax into the comfort of the walking shoes.

7. You're stuffed.

You should wait an hour or two after a meal to begin an aerobic workout; otherwise circulation will be diverted from your digestive track just when it needs oxygenated blood to process the meal. As you walk, the muscles of the lower extremities will take circulation away from the autonomic muscles of the stomach, sometimes causing a bloated or cramped sensation.

But after you've given that big meal a chance to settle, by all means take a walk! By stimulating the abdominal muscles, walking speeds up digestion, keeps the bowels regular, and prevents constipation. It also encourages the muscles to burn the fats circulating in the blood, rather than blood sugar, helping you burn up some of those calories. Your basal metabolism—the rate at which your body ordinarily burns energy—increases from 14 to 18 percent after walking. And your body continues to work more efficiently for many hours after your walk, a boon to those who want to lose weight or simply avoid gaining.

Once your metabolic engine is warmed up by walking, it continues to burn more energy for the next 6 hours. Scientists estimate this increased calorie burning can result in an extra 4 to 5 pounds lost in a year.

8. You don't want to get heart disease.

Over the last forty years, numerous studies have shown that active people have fewer heart attacks than those who don't exercise. One reason for this is that exercise strengthens the heart's ability to pump and helps it withstand stress. The aerobically fit heart pumps more oxygen and blood—in essence, works more efficiently. Each heartbeat pumps out more blood; thus fewer beats a minute are needed to pump the same blood volume. This allows a slower resting heart rate and lower blood pressure.

At the same time, walking is strengthening your muscles and lungs and their ability to use oxygen efficiently. This means your heart doesn't have to work so hard to feed all the blood vessels. The aerobically fit body is thus able to work harder and longer with less fatigue and less dangerous strain.

Some exercise fanatics have scoffed at walking as a wimpy exercise that doesn't do much to increase aerobic capacity. But new studies show that walking is "aerobic enough." Although walking does not speed up the heart as much as running or aerobic dance, a brisk walk does raise the heart rate to "training threshold" for the vast majority of adults. And training threshold is the level that conditions the cardiovascular system to optimum health.

9. You're nervous and upset, and you have a good reason.

There are times in every adult's life when problems and hassles are really overwhelming. Perhaps a loved one is ill. Or you've just made a terrible mistake.

I'm not going to tell you that you can walk such problems away. But walking will help you keep yourself in the best possible shape for coping with "the slings and arrows of outrageous fortune." It's not selfish to take an hour out of even the most pressured day to care for yourself. It may be the best thing you can do for others. You'll be able to think more clearly and handle your emotions better when you come back.

10. You have your period.

Or you're in the premenstrual phase and feel bloated and irritable. Much of the discomfort of the end of the menstrual cycle stems from the fact that your tissues retain more water than usual. This can cause painful breasts, swollen ankles, a sense of being bloated, and irritability stemming from too much water in the tissues of the brain.

By speeding up your metabolism, walking serves as a diuretic, increasing the elimination of excess water. Not only will you feel better if you take a walk now, but a regular walking program may virtually eliminate premenstrual and menstrual discomfort.

11. You're a patriotic American concerned with the future of your country.

Everyone knows that our nation's health-care costs are skyrocketing to the point that they threaten our economic prosperity. But not everyone realizes there's something individuals can do about it. These days, keeping fit and healthy is a patriotic duty. Not only will you and your family be happier if you seldom need to use your medical insurance or Medicare benefits, but the whole nation will benefit.

12. You love your family.

Setting a good example for your children, spouse, or parents is a great way to express that love. Don't tell them to get out and exercise, just do it yourself. They'll see your enthusiasm and how refreshed and high-spirited you appear when you get back. It may take months, or even years, before your example actually inspires them, but sooner or later it will. Children of parents who exercise naturally fold activity into their daily schedule when they get older. Even elderly parents can be inspired to do some walking by your example.

13. Your sex drive is flagging.

Lack of interest in sex has become the number-one sexual problem in America. No wonder. We're all so busy working and organizing demanding leisure-time activities that there's no pause, no empty time in our lives for our basic biological urges to make themselves heard. We miss too many opportunities to express our desire and love in that most basic act.

Walking tall and sucking in the abdomen stimulates the sexual organs by increasing blood circulation to the area. Walking increases your awareness of your body and its basic beauty. Allowing your thoughts to drift into sexual fantasy as you walk can aid the process. You and your partner will be pleased by a slow, undramatic, but definite increase in sexual interest.

14. You're not good at higher mathematics.

Many reluctant exercisers have thrown in the towel in annoyance when instructors have insisted they count their pulse and use arcane formulas to measure their progress. An exercise laboratory recently came up with the following "simple" formula to measure aerobic capacity after a 1-mile walk:

VO 2 max (mL/kg/min) = 132.853 [0.0769 × (body weight in pounds)] [0.3877 × (age in years)] + (6.3150 × SEX) (3.2649 × T) (0.1565 × HR)

The good news is that you don't have to use this formula to follow the Walk It Off! program. You don't even have to take your pulse! If you walk fast enough to feel slightly out of breath after 20 minutes, you're doing well. Other signs that you're increasing your aerobic capacity are flushed skin and the ability to walk farther and faster over a period of weeks. A tingling, itching sensation in your legs, arms, or chest is another positive sign. This occurs because your heart rate is speeding up and opening up (dilating) the blood vessels. They press against the superficial nerves in your skin and cause the tingling sensation.

One sure way to make sure you don't overdo it: never move so fast that you can't speak easily as you walk.

15. You want to stay "forever young."

Though physical changes are a natural part of the aging process, inactivity can make you older quicker. Many of the aches, pains, and ailments we think of as connected to old age are, in fact, due to a lack of fitness, what geriatric expert Robert Butler, M.D., calls "the voluntary shuffling of the elderly."Even osteoporosis—the loss of bone density that causes some old people to grow shorter and suffer bone breaks—has been shown to be preventable by exercise.

Many of the afflictions of old age, such as memory loss, confusion, incontinence, poor blood circulation, joint pain and joint locking in arthritis, muscle weakness, and trouble moving around, can be prevented by walking—and even reversed by walking once they've set in. In one study, people between the ages of 70 and 86 increased their aerobic capacity by 13 percent by following a walking program for just twelve weeks. That's the difference between feeling pooped from a brief shopping trip and having enough energy to enjoy an all-day family party.

> *Middle-aged adults who are active* tend to be in a much better mood than their more sedentary counterparts. Long-term exercise is also associated with higher self-esteem.

As far as longevity is concerned, "the ideal exercise in every respect is walking," says Dr. Henry A. Solomon of Cornell University Medical Center in New York. In a large-scale study of Harvard graduates, the beneficial effects of go-slow, moderate exercise on the life span were clear. Men who walked briskly for 9 or more miles a week (enough to burn off at least 900 calories) had a 21 percent lower risk of death than those who walked less than 3 miles a week.

The longest lives were seen in men who did about 35 miles of brisk walking a week and burned at least 3,500 calories. But, interestingly, those who did more than that level of exercise actually had a higher death rate than their more moderate classmates. The Walk It Off! program is designed to put you right on target for the maximum benefits of exercise on your life span.

An okay from the doctor is advisable for any older person who hasn't exercised before. Don't be surprised, though, if your doctor gives a blessing to the idea. Walking is the medicine doctors really prescribe most!

5

The Feelings

How do couch potatoes, slouches, and the hopelessly unathletic manage to turn themselves into walkers? That's a question I always ask the audiences at the corporate wellness programs where I'm invited back year after year. My veteran walkers usually pinpoint the same success secret: "I finally just made up my mind to do it, and then it was easy."

I think this response is true enough—as far as it goes. But it skips over the very real and prolonged struggle that most of us go through *before* we can make up our minds to do it.

When I began experimenting with my own walking routine I was often tempted to say to myself, loudly and firmly, "Okay, this is it, I've decided, I'm going to walk 45 minutes a day, five times a week, for the rest of my life." But each time a small, cynical voice answered: "Oh, sure you will, just like you succeeded with tennis and bike riding. You've always been a short, chubby, unathletic person. A tiger can't change her stripes!"

In the hopes of resolving this internal conflict, I began to research what is known scientifically about how people manage to make changes in their life-styles. I read loads of studies and articles, and called up some of the important public health researchers who did them.

What I learned is that there are two important factors that separate the exercise doers from the dropouts. One is what researchers call self-efficacy—the *learned* self-confidence that you can perform a specific behavior (like walking) under specific conditions (every morning before breakfast). And the other is social support—the family members, coworkers, and neighbors who cheer you on your way.

Women walk faster than men . . . and cover more territory, says a researcher who spent years observing pedestrians in Lincoln, Nebraska. In a study of 200 adults, he clocked women at an average rate of 256 feet per minute, while men walked at 245 feet per minute.

This information proved very valuable to me as I worked to create a walking habit. For one thing, I was glad to learn that it wasn't simply a matter of "willpower," that grit-your-teeth-and-do-it-even-if-it-hurts attitude that I seem to have been born without.

"We find that it's persistence, not willpower, that gets people to change their behavior," says public health researcher Victor J. Strecher, Ph.D., of the University of North Carolina. "You engage in behaviors that you think you can do in the first place. And if you think that you can do them, you're more likely to *persist* in trying to change."

We are not born with either the self-efficacy or the social support that allows us to change our habits. But we all do have the power to create our own sense of efficacy, or power, over our life-styles, and to develop a social support system that will help us on our way.

This chapter is designed to help you build up your personal and social sense of power. It will give you the tools for changing your life-style. These tools can help you acquire a walking habit, and then go on to make other changes you may wish in your life-style—

such as losing weight, improving your social life, or giving up negative addictions.

I Think I Can, I Think I Can . . .

Jim M. and Rusty G. met when they were roommates in the hospital, both recovering from serious heart attacks. When they were released, they received the same advice from their doctors: lose weight, reduce cholesterol intake, and get some exercise. The two men kept in touch, and a few months after their heart attacks they met to compare notes.

Jim M. had lost 7 pounds, switched to low-fat milk, given up french fries, and gotten into the new habit of walking to and from work each day. He looked good, he felt great, and he was very proud of himself.

On-the-job exercise varies greatly with occupation. Factory workers, commodities runners, and messengers walk the most—over 6 miles a day. Nurses, bank workers, and home-makers walk more than 4 miles during their work days. But dental hygienists, newspaper editors, and law clerks log in under 3 miles a day.

Rusty G. had left the hospital with equally good intentions. He had sworn off cake and ice cream, but found himself cheating regularly and actually gained a few pounds. He went jogging a few times, but never managed to do it regularly. "I'm just not the health type," Rusty told Jim. "I can't control myself."

Jim was not convinced that Rusty's problem lay in his "type" or "character." "I knew I could follow the doctor's orders because I had practice doing it," he told Rusty. "Four years ago I gave up smoking. That was really hard, and I figured if I could do that, I could certainly walk to work every day. You must have changed some habits in your lifetime. You supervise a huge warehouse; surely you had to overcome some problems along the way.''

After some thought, Rusty recalled that when he started as a supervisor he used to get furiously angry and scream at any employee who came in late. But over the years he had trained himself not to yell or even feel angry. Instead, he took the worker aside and explained how his lateness had created a burden for his co-workers, a tactic that did much more to curb the problem.

''Well, if you could learn to control your anger, you can certainly learn to take a walk every day,'' said Jim. And, in fact, Rusty did manage to make the desired changes in his life-style. He thought back to the techniques he had used years before to learn to control his temper and used those same strengths to guide himself into an exercise and diet routine.

''The ability to change health habits takes a collection of skills you acquire over a long period of time,'' says Dr. Strecher. ''People who have developed self-efficacy are more likely to tackle challenges like changing eating habits or quitting smoking, and they're more likely to succeed.''

Interestingly, Strecher's research shows that people build their self-confidence through a series of half steps, sidesteps, and even back steps. ''In our addiction clinics, we find the average person fails four times before he succeeds. By the time people make it, they've learned from their previous lapses. They know how to handle situations that in the past made them reach for a cigarette, or a drink, or cocaine.''

So success can be built on past failures, slips, lapses, and relapses, as long as these are seen as opportunities to improve, not reasons to give up. (See Chapter 16 for tips on recovering from lapses.) In fact, it's this trial-and-error process that encourages the growth of what scientists call self-efficacy and what the rest of us call self-confidence and sheer persistence, the ''I think I can, I think I can'' pluckiness of the locomotive in the children's story *The Little Engine That Could.* Self-efficacy is not an inborn condition, but rather something we can learn from the right set of experiences.

Here are some mental exercises designed to help you tap in to what you already know about changing your life-style.

Exercise 1

Identify a successful experience you've had with change:

_____ gave up smoking
_____ cut down on alcohol consumption
_____ stopped biting fingernails or sucking thumb
_____ developed neater habits
_____ changed an eating habit
_____ changed dating or sexual habits
_____ learned to control anger
_____ started sleeping regular hours
_____ learned to save money
_____ began to wear a seatbelt
_____ learned to be more patient
_____ stopped oversleeping in the morning
_____ learned to work more efficiently
_____ began to use condoms during sexual intercourse
_____ learned to get along better with your spouse
_____ stopped combining drinking with driving
_____ became more understanding of your parents
_____ eliminated unhealthy foods
_____ started a more careful tooth cleaning routine

_____

Exercise 2

Of those checked, choose the one change experience that was most difficult for you and answer the following questions about your experience. If you've made two or more important life-style changes, do this exercise separately for each one.

What prompted the decision to change: _____

_____

Was it a gradual or sudden change? _____

How long did you think about changing before you did it? ____

Did you have any lapses or failures after you started? _____

What did you do when you failed? _____

What was the worst problem you had in making the change? __

How did you solve the problem? _____

Did you reward yourself for changing? _____

Did you model your change after another person? _____

How did you remember to stick to your new habit? _____

Were you afraid of failing? _____

Did you keep a record of your progress? _____

Did you tell other people about the decision? Who? _____

Which people were helpful in leading you to change? How did they help? _____

Note: Not all of these questions are equally relevant to each experience you've had in changing habits. But your answers to at least some of the above will be relevant to your work at gaining a walking habit. Go back over your answers and put a star next to each of the ones that you think you might be able to apply to walking.

Forewarned Is Forearmed

In the following exercise, I want you to anticipate all the kinds of problems you're likely to face as you try to integrate walking into your everyday routine. The point of this is not to discourage you, but to help you devise a strategy for dealing with each potential problem *in advance* so that it doesn't defeat you.

Exercise 3

Which of the following problems are you likely to encounter?

1. _____ I feel too tired to walk.
2. _____ The telephone rings just as I'm leaving for my walk.
3. _____ My legs and feet ache.
4. _____ I feel discouraged because I didn't do it yesterday.
5. _____ The weather is bad: rain, cold, heat.
6. _____ My child or spouse interferes with my schedule.
7. _____ I oversleep.
8. _____ I have a lunch engagement at the time I'd planned to walk.
9. _____ I overeat and then feel too fat to walk.
10. _____ I forget.
11. _____ I put it off.
12. _____ I am bored with the routine.
13. _____ I'm lazy.

Now we need to draw up a battle-plan for defeating the foes of walking. I have some strategies for overcoming the walking enemies listed above, but don't just take my word for it. Rather, read what I have to say, recall your own personal experiences from Exercise 1, and come up with your own remedy for each of your potential walking problems.

1. I feel too tired to walk.

My strategy on days when I'm feeling really tired is to allow myself a 5-minute "power rest." I take off my shoes and lie down on the couch, bed, or even the carpeted floor of my office with a pillow under my head. I note the time and give myself permission to relax totally for 5 minutes. If I think I might actually fall asleep, I set an alarm clock.

Then after 5 minutes, I get up slowly and begin my stretching routine. I tell myself I'll go out and walk briskly for 5 minutes. Then if I still feel really tired and don't feel like continuing, I'll turn around and come home. Two times I actually did return home after a 5-minute walk: it turned out I was coming down with an illness and did, indeed, need rest more than exercise. Every other time (and there have been dozens and dozens) I've ended up finishing my walk and reenergizing myself for the day ahead.

Stop for a moment and imagine yourself really very tired. What will you do if you feel this way when you've scheduled your walk?

2. The telephone rings just as I'm leaving for my walk.

This happens to me so often that I've developed several strategies for dealing with it. If my husband or one of my children is home, I'll yell, "Tell whoever it is I'm out," and race out the door. If not, I let my answering machine take the call. If I'm feeling very strong-willed, I won't even listen as the message is recorded so I won't be tempted to pick up the call. But if I think it might be an emergency, I'll listen, and I'll pick it up only if it is. Sometimes I just answer the phone automatically, and many's the time I've "wakened up" 15 minutes later to realize I've talked away my precious walking time. Now I'm careful to start the conversation by saying, "Oh, I'm just going out the door for my walk. When can I call you back?"

Who's likely to call you at the wrong minute? Rehearse a couple of ways you can handle the problem.

3. My legs and feet ache.

If you've just started walking regularly and your legs or feet ache, be sure to stretch slowly and carefully before you begin *and* to stretch again on your return home. However, if you've been walking for some time and still have this problem, turn to Chapter 12 and read up on the causes of aching muscles and feet. It may be that your next walk should be to a physician's or podiatrist's office.

4. I feel discouraged because I didn't do it yesterday.

This is one of the hardest walking obstacles for me personally to overcome. As soon as I miss a day, especially if I didn't really have a good reason, I begin to doubt my ability to stick with the program.

This is really the time to make a strong effort to turn your thinking around. Review your personal walking goals and reread the motivating facts in Chapter 4. Glance through your Walker's Log, and instead of focusing on yesterday's defeat, think about the times you did succeed in walking. And while you're thinking, get into your walking clothes and start stretching.

5. The weather is bad: rain, cold, heat.

Planning where to walk in bad weather is one of the most important things you can do to help yourself establish a walking habit. Almost everyone has access to an indoor shopping mall that is kept pleasantly dry and at a moderate temperature all year round. All the better if you can find one indoor walking spot near your home and another near your office.

You may need to change the time of day of your usual walk when the weather is bad. If you can't walk to the train in the morning, for example, you might have to wait until early evening to find time to get to a shopping mall. Plan in advance how you'll handle this so the poor weather doesn't throw you.

6. My child or spouse interferes with my schedule.

Sometimes, of course, the walking schedule will have to bend if your child, your spouse, or even the next-door neighbor desperately needs your attention just as you're ready to leave the house. But if this becomes a pattern, it's time to sit down and talk about it (after you come back from your walk).

The problem, however, may be more in your mind than in the interferers. Are you afraid that your loved ones really can't do without you for even an hour a day? If so, remember that only when you're at your personal best—physically fit, energetic, and happy—can you deliver the best care and love to them. If you have trouble getting to walk for your own sake, do it for their sakes!

7. I oversleep.

Since I usually walk in the morning, before breakfast, oversleeping is a problem I have from time to time. Sometimes I forget to set my alarm. Sometimes I manage to ignore it when it goes off. And sometimes I say the hell with it and turn it off and grab an extra 30 minutes of sleep.

If this is a chronic problem for you, then it may be that early morning is not the ideal time for you to walk. Try switching to a lunchtime or early-evening schedule. But if it just happens once in a while, as it does for me, it's probably best to forgive yourself. Make sure you do walk at some time during the day you overslept, and reinstate your morning habit the next day.

8. I have a lunch engagement at the time I'd planned to walk.

If you plan to walk during your lunch break, you need to consider how to ward off competitors for your time. What if your boss makes a snide remark that everyone else eats at his or her desk and keeps working, while you trot around the block? What if your usual lunch date gets miffed at the change? Will you miss the socializing at lunchtime?

All of these are solvable problems, but you need to think out in advance how you'll handle them. For example, remarks about how your lunchtime walk is doubling your energy and productivity in the afternoon are apt to get the boss on your side. You can invite your usual lunch partner to become your walking partner. And don't hesitate to suggest a walk first to anyone who invites you to lunch. The nation is full of budding walkers these days—people who are grateful for any chance to reinforce their habit.

9. I overeat and then feel too fat to walk.

I call this my "Monday-morning problem," because it's usually over the weekends that I grow hazy about my healthy eating plan and give in to various temptations. Then on Monday morning I wake up feeling bloated and discouraged and hop on the scale to have my worse fears confirmed. The negative voice inside begins to mutter: What's the use? You're so fat anyway, what's a 60-minute walk going to do?

I've learned to defeat the Monday-morning blues through a couple of sneaky tactics. First, I never weigh myself on Monday. Tuesday's soon enough, and if I'm back to my healthy eating habits all day Monday, the Tuesday-morning verdict might not be that bad.

Then I put on my spiffiest walking outfit, and even add a little lipstick and mascara before I do my stretching and HAPPY routines in front of the mirror. When I'm feeling my worst, I make a special effort to look my best.

What tactics will you use to get yourself going on "the morning after"? Think it through and the overweight blues won't defeat you.

10. I forget.

This doesn't happen much to me, but it does happen to a friend of mine. Kerry H., who owns a retail office supply store, is one of those people who always starts his day making a careful list of things to do, organizes the list into priority order, slips it under the blotter on his desk, and never so much as glances at the list for the rest of the day. Small wonder he doesn't always remember to do the things that are on it!

If you're a "forgetter," it's especially important to take your walk at the same time each day whenever possible. Ingrained routines do not even have to be remembered; the body goes through them on automatic pilot.

Another tactic is to find a reliable walking partner to serve as your prompter. Kerry takes his walk with a man from a neighboring business. The partner simply shows up at Kerry's store at 1:00 p.m. every day, and although Kerry sometimes stares at him blankly, wondering why he's there, the partner is happy to remind him it's time for their daily walk.

11. I put it off.

Procrastination is one of America's favorite indoor sports. The game goes like this. You wake up in the morning, consider taking a walk, but then think, oh, it's still a little chilly out, the weather will be pleasanter later on. Then at noon, the thought of walking crosses your mind again, but you've got errands to run and calls to make, and by the time you look up, it's 5:30 p.m. You could walk halfway home and then catch the bus, but you feel draggy and tired, and you decide to walk after dinner instead. By 8:00 at night you're deeply engrossed in a favorite TV program. By 10:00, when the program is over, you decide it's too late, too chilly, and too dangerous to go out on the street.

It took only a few days like the one I just described to make me realize that if I didn't walk first thing in the morning, I'd never manage to squeeze it in. If you find yourself procrastinating, you're probably giving yourself too much freedom. Choose a walking time, and stick to it.

12. I am bored with the routine.

Some people love routine; they prefer to do the same activities, in the same order, in the same way, day after day. Once these people decide on a convenient slot for fitting in their walking time, they have little trouble sticking to it.

Other people love novelty and change. Doing the same thing even a few days in a row makes them feel fidgety, restless, buried alive. If you're one of those, you need to use your restless imagination to make each day's walk a new experience. I believe it's best *not* to vary the time of day that you walk, because this works against the very habit-forming mechanisms you're trying to instill. But there's no harm at all in varying your walking route. No two walks need be in the same direction. Choose a different path, a different track, and different companions as often as you like.

13. I'm lazy.

I'd be surprised if there were any readers who did not check laziness as a potential problem. One of the negative effects of the fitness movement was that it convinced those of us who were left behind that we were "lazy."

Laziness can actually be a healthy trait. In our fast-paced lifestyles, it's often a form of self-protection. The world may be screaming that we "must" do a thousand tasks, but our inner selves are saying "Help," "I won't," or "I can't." So when I realize I'm feeling lazy I don't berate myself. I say, "Oh, poor thing, you've really been doing too much, no wonder you feel lazy."

Then I set up a situation in which going for a walk is the lesser of two evils. Well, I think, I'm feeling kind of lazy but I can't afford to do nothing. So, I can either balance my checkbook now (a long-overdue activity) or go for a walk. Or I can straighten up the kitchen and call my mother, or go for a walk.

If you're feeling lazy, don't fight it. Just make taking a walk the most lazy thing you're allowed to do.

Getting By with a Little Help from Your Friends

Anyone who's successfully held down a job, raised a child, financed a house, or graduated from school knows that help from others is part of every individual's success story. Perhaps your spouse makes sure you get up in time to get to work or takes over when you're too tense to deal with a child. Maybe your parents lent you money for a down payment for a house or helped you finance your education. Or you may have friends who encouraged you to apply for a desirable job or checked the spelling on your application.

Aristotle was so fond of walking while he reasoned that the philosophers who followed his teachings are called the Peripatetics—"those who walk about."

Help like this does not diminish the individual's achievement. We're all social animals, and other people's good opinions do matter to us. So while it's probably *possible* to develop a walking habit without any help from anyone, it's a lot easier and pleasanter to use all the help you can find.

"Our need for each other is a virtue to be celebrated rather than an obstacle to be overcome," says psychologist Judd Allen, who has designed corporate wellness programs for such business giants as Johnson & Johnson. "It's normal not to be able to maintain a good health habit unless you have a supportive environment. Support group programs are very helpful, but they don't last a lifetime." Each individual needs to find support and encouragement from his family, friends, and colleagues at work—the people he normally encounters on a daily basis—or new people, added to his life, for the sole purpose of supporting the walking habit. The following exercise should help you sniff out the people who'll help or hinder you in your new fitness campaign.

Exercise 4

List the people you see or talk to frequently and consider what kind of support you can expect to get from them for your walking habit. If possible, include people from work, the neighborhood, and your family. I'm allowing space for you to rate the support you expect to receive from ten people, but you may not be able to think of ten right now. However, you can add people to the list as you encounter them.

1. (person's name) _____
_____ may become a walking partner
_____ will not walk, but may strongly encourage me
_____ can be taught to encourage me
_____ will remain neutral
_____ is likely to discourage me

2. (person's name) _____
_____ may become a walking partner
_____ will not walk, but may strongly encourage me
_____ can be taught to encourage me
_____ will remain neutral
_____ is likely to discourage me

3. (person's name) _____
_____ may become a walking partner
_____ will not walk, but may strongly encourage me
_____ can be taught to encourage me
_____ will remain neutral
_____ is likely to discourage me

4. (person's name) _____
_____ may become a walking partner
_____ will not walk, but may strongly encourage me
_____ can be taught to encourage me
_____ will remain neutral
_____ is likely to discourage me

5. (person's name) _____

    _____ may become a walking partner
    _____ will not walk, but may strongly encourage me
    _____ can be taught to encourage me
    _____ will remain neutral
    _____ is likely to discourage me

6. (person's name) _____

    _____ may become a walking partner
    _____ will not walk, but may strongly encourage me
    _____ can be taught to encourage me
    _____ will remain neutral
    _____ is likely to discourage me

7. (person's name) _____

    _____ may become a walking partner
    _____ will not walk, but may strongly encourage me
    _____ can be taught to encourage me
    _____ will remain neutral
    _____ is likely to discourage me

8. (person's name) _____

    _____ may become a walking partner
    _____ will not walk, but may strongly encourage me
    _____ can be taught to encourage me
    _____ will remain neutral
    _____ is likely to discourage me

9. (person's name) _____

    _____ may become a walking partner
    _____ will not walk, but may strongly encourage me
    _____ can be taught to encourage me
    _____ will remain neutral
    _____ is likely to discourage me

10. (person's name) ————————————————————

    ———— may become a walking partner

    ———— will not walk, but may strongly encourage me

    ———— can be taught to encourage me

    ———— will remain neutral

    ———— is likely to discourage me

Changing Enemies into Friends

Before you decide to file for divorce, end a friendship, or disown a parent based on the preceding exercise, it's important to remember that some people are naturally good at giving encouragement, while others need to be taught now. It's worth at least trying to teach those around you how to give the support you need. If after a few lessons they prove unteachable, then give up. And, as much as possible, avoid talking about your walking program to people who are likely to discourage you or put you down.

In general, according to the research of Victor Strecher, women are better than men at giving support and enhancing each other's self-efficacy. Many men tend to poke fun at each other, and at their female friends' attempts to change and improve.

"I've seen men who think they're supporting their wives' attempts to exercise by calling them 'fatty,' " says Strecher. "They think that insults and humiliation will goad their wives into action. But, in fact, it has the opposite effect—the women just give up."

Anyone who attempts to "manhandle" you into changing should be told calmly and firmly that his or her approach needs changing. "I know you don't mean to be discouraging, but it's more helpful if you don't poke fun at my figure when I'm trying to start a new program." If your critic asks, "What should I say?" have your answer ready.

Here are some sample actions and supportive remarks that any willing friend or relative can learn to make:

Remind you of past successes. "Remember the time you took aer-obics for five weeks? You stuck to that. I bet you can walk every day for ten weeks this time around."

Go with you. A friend who walks along with you every once in a while can bolster your routine. He or she doesn't have to make a steady commitment to be a walking partner.

Compliment your efforts. "Oh, you're in your walking suit—that's a good start." Or "Didn't you walk yesterday, too? You're really getting into this." Or "You look so pink and alive after your walk."

Remind you of your goals. "You said you were going to go out for a walk instead of getting nervous worrying . . . and here you are doing it!" Or "I think walking is making you look thinner, even if you haven't lost weight yet."

Finding New Walking Friends

I met Lila at my neighborhood library. She was wearing a warm-up suit, and so was I, so I used that as a conversation-starter. She turned out to be a warm, animated woman, in her mid-70s, who had recently begun a morning walking routine in the park. After finding that she lived not far from my building, I took the plunge and offered to be her walking partner.

Lila was thrilled with the invitation. She lived alone and was quite anxious for companionship. For me she was also the ideal partner. She was reliable and showed up every morning on time, which made me redouble my efforts to get out on time, too. She didn't talk too much while we walked, so I could enjoy some mental privacy. And, to tell the truth, she was not so young, or so slim, or so good-looking that she made me feel inferior. (At this time I was 60 pounds overweight and most people I met *did* make me feel inferior.)

For a couple of years, until she moved to another state, Lila was able to give me a kind of gentle support and companionship that neither my husband, my children, my parents, nor my colleagues could. After Lila moved, I joined the Walking Association of New York and frequently engage in group walks in the park on Sundays. I enjoy talking to the other walkers and feel that it reinforces my desire to keep up the habit. And I'm also hoping to run into another Lila, someone who lives close by and is interested in walking on the same schedule.

If your evaluation of your close friends and family members has not produced a walking companion, consider seeking one out. A good tactic is to put a notice on local bulletin boards at exercise studios, schools, tennis courts, or an Overeaters Anonymous or Alcoholics Anonymous group.

Another good place to make contacts is at any health or wellness program sponsored by your workplace. These are becoming increasingly common. Over half of large companies, and 15 percent of smaller ones, now sponsor some kind of fitness program, according to a January 1989 study published in the *American Journal of Public Health*. These programs are often started by a CEO who has just had a heart attack or been treated for alcoholism and wants to spread the good health information he or she has learned.

If there's no fitness program at your workplace, consider rounding up a few like-minded colleagues and starting one. It doesn't take a megacorporation with megabucks to get one started.

Last year, for example, the city of Portland, Oregon, organized a "Play for Health" program during the month of March—a health fair that included walks, lectures, cooking demonstrations, cholesterol testing, and field trips. The program was free to the community, and many smaller employers—who make up the bulk of the Portland workforce—sent company teams. "We used it as an opportunity to spur each other on," reports Evelyn Whitlock, M.D., who cochaired "Play for Health." "Some of us who were active already were able to use our motivation to encourage others to take steps on their own behalf. Nobody operates in a vacuum. None of us are superheros who can do it on their own. Making behavior changes is one of the hardest things people do; a supportive environment makes it possible."

6

The Rewards

The day I proudly realized I'd succeeded in walking five mornings a week for four straight weeks, I decided I deserved a treat. My first thought was food—a hot fudge sundae, a box of chocolate truffles. But it seemed rather foolish to use fattening food as a reward for doing something positive for my health. My thoughts then turned to silk scarves, gold earrings, and designer shoes, but our family finances were not currently fit for such extravagances. Anyway, I wanted a *real* reward, not a temporary one that would make me feel sorry the next time I got on the scale or looked at my bank balance.

All the way to work that morning I tried to finish the sentence "The reward I'd really like is . . ." Nothing much suggested itself until the end of the day, when my last patient canceled his appointment. Usually, when that happens I rush home early and delve into the waiting household chores. But this time, I recognized the cancellation as an opportunity for fun. I grabbed a newspaper, checked the schedule, and took myself out to a neighborhood movie.

I'll never forget how strange and delicious it felt entering the dark theater all alone. I bought popcorn (no butter) and a diet soda and sat in the mostly empty theater feeling all the thrilling pleasure of a child playing hooky from school. The movie was great, and the whole experience left me feeling independent, successful, and happy for days. So happy, in fact, that I noticed I was particularly sweet to my husband, patient with my children, kind to my parents, and attentive to my patients.

The experience taught me two things. First, I had been so busy fulfilling my obligations to other people that I often forgot to do the simple things that make me feel happy. And, second, when I took the time to please myself, it had a ripple effect and ended up pleasing those that I cared about, too. Since then, I've tried to reward myself for walking on a daily basis, and to celebrate my walking "milestones" (six months with the program; graduating to the intermediate level, and so on) with a bigger treat.

Yes, I know I've been saying all along that walking is its own reward—that just doing it will make you feel good. But true as this is, walkers also deserve other kinds of rewards for sticking with the program. After all, we're taking good care of ourselves. And the effort we put into protecting our physical and mental health rewards those around us and society as a whole. So why not rechannel some of that positive energy back into our own lives by rewarding ourselves for doing well? One good turn deserves another!

The idea of rewarding yourself for exercising may make you feel uncomfortable. In general, doing things for your health is not rewarded in our society. Most workplaces will give you sick days and help pay doctor's bills, but they don't reward you for staying well and coming to work every day, points out corporate health consultant Judd Allen. Your boss may bring in a big box of doughnuts or take the staff out for a drink after a difficult project is completed. But this type of reward certainly can't be carried over to walking— it would work against your health goals. Judd Allen has convinced some corporations to give "well" days to workers who don't take sick time and bonuses to all employees if health insurance costs go down. He believes if you want to encourage good behavior, you must reward it.

I'd like to convince you to award yourself a series of bonuses, "me breaks," and well days. It may feel a bit awkward at first. You may feel "selfish" allowing yourself even such minor treats as lying down for a half-hour nap or taking a long soak in the tub with the radio on. But these treats refresh the spirit and renew your will to keep up with your walking. And they'll make you a pleasanter person to be around.

You're a walker now, so you're entitled to do other things that are good for you too. But beware. This is not a "quick fix" program. The rewards, like the walking program, are meant to produce long-range changes. That means that you'll soon feel "entitled" to the small pleasures you set up as daily and milestone rewards. Feeling good is habit-forming!

The 15-Minute "Me" Break

Most of us are not used to giving ourselves constructive rewards. After an exhausting day's work we might reach for a martini, or turn on the television and flip the channels—but these are not real rewards. Rather, they're a flight from the day, an attempt to turn off the mental tape that keeps rerunning thoughts of "what I should have said" and "what I forgot to do."

Giving yourself a small reward every time you succeed in walking is not like these attempts to escape the stress of the workday. First of all, it's much more positive. You're doing something nice for yourself because you've just done something else nice for yourself. And, second of all, it's an open claim for a little happiness. It says, "I felt good while I was walking, and now I want to feel good for another 15 minutes. What can I do to prolong the feeling?"

Let's face it—easy and pleasurable as walking is, it still takes discipline and effort to develop a walking habit. It means creating a basic change in your daily routine, adding one more thing to the "must do" and "must remember" list. As far as I'm concerned, you deserve a medal every time you do it!

But what kind of medal? We all respond to different pleasures. If you're the parent of two children under 6, 15 minutes of uninterrupted time is a tremendous rarity and reward, and it doesn't matter if you spend it soaking in the tub, gazing out the window, or reading the newspaper. But if you live alone and see few people, you're apt to crave company more than solitude; for you, 15 minutes spent talking to an interesting neighbor might be an excellent post-walk reward.

The following exercise is designed to help you explore what kind of "me break" you'd enjoy. Go through this list and check all the rewards listed that appeal to you.

Exercise 1

Check the things you might enjoy doing:

_____ a 15-minute nap

_____ sitting and staring out the window for 15 minutes

_____ calling someone you enjoy talking to:

_____(name)

_____ not picking up the telephone when it rings

_____ buying and reading a magazine

_____ listening to the radio for 15 minutes

_____ taking a 15-minute bubble bath

_____ inviting a neighbor over for a quick cup of coffee

_____ giving yourself a manicure

_____ taking the time to prepare one of your own favorite dishes

_____ watching an interesting television program that you often miss

_____ shaving *slowly*, applying pre-shave and after-shave lotions

_____ taking a bike ride

_____ driving to a nearby scenic area and watching the sunset

_____ writing a letter to a friend, or a "letter to the editor" of your local newspaper

_____ rubbing body cream all over your skin

_____ reading the instruction manual of a new electronic device
_____ hosing down the car
_____ cleaning out a silverware drawer

Choosing Rewards

Choose rewards for the next three times you walk. You may choose some of those on the list above, or make up your own. The rewards can be "treats," or, like cleaning out a silverware drawer or taking a long-overdue book back to the library, they can be rewards in the sense of taking care of something that's been nagging at you and preventing you from feeling good. Sometimes my reward is calling a sick relative I've felt guilty about neglecting, or ringing the bell of an elderly neighbor just to chat or offer assistance. Sometimes, doing good for others is the best way to make yourself feel good!

Reward 1: _____

Reward 2: _____

Reward 3: _____

Now that you have an inkling about what types of rewards appeal to you, make sure that you implement them! If you're very rushed after your walk, it's okay to give yourself an IOU. For example, if you walk in the morning and then have to rush off to work, you can make a date with yourself to listen to music for 15 minutes during the evening and enlist your spouse in keeping the children out of your way, or answering the phone and taking messages, during that time period.

It's not necessary to explain to other people exactly what you're doing with your walking rewards. You can just tell your spouse you're taking a "stress break" or practicing meditation. But do be sure to acknowledge to yourself what the reward is for. Something simple like thinking, "Ah, now I'm going to lie down for 15 minutes; I deserve it; I got out and walked today even though it was drizzling and I was feeling kind of down." Or "I'm going to call my friend for a chat now and reward myself and her with how cheerful I feel after my walk."

Milestone Celebrations

Birthday and anniversary celebrations are, of course, very popular, though, to my mind, they always have an edge of sadness. They mark the passage of time and emphasize that we're one year older.

Walking celebrations are a bit different. They celebrate accomplishment (moving from the beginning to the intermediate walking program, for example) and sticking to the program for a substantial time. I like to celebrate at least once each month. Usually on the first of the month, when I start a new page in my Walker's Log, I like to look back at the past month to see what I've accomplished. If I've done well and stuck to my goals whenever possible, I plan a little anniversary celebration for myself.

At times, I've celebrated all by myself. I have a very hectic lifestyle, and I often feel pulled in many different directions by the important people in my life: my patients, my office staff, my husband, my daughters, my parents, and my friends. So for me, solitude is a treasured reward.

But at other times, I've arranged celebrations to include my walking supporters. Once I invited my friend Lila, who walked with me every morning for months, to accompany me for what was the first massage of both of our lives. It was a new and very pleasurable reward, and it felt less strange because we did it together. Another time I invited a friend who had always cheered my walking program to join me for a gourmet, but low-calorie, spa lunch that had just been instituted by a New York hotel. We raised our glasses of sparkling water and toasted each other's efforts to stay healthy and sane amid the turmoil of careers and family life.

What's the right kind of celebration for you once you've reached a walking milestone? Try to celebrate in a way that fills some void or lack in your life. I've noticed that people usually suffer from one of two types of voids. Either they've got too little to do, and find their lives unstimulating, or they've got too much to do and find their lives overloaded. If you're among the understimulated, choose a celebration that gets you out among people and new ideas. If you're among the overloaded, choose a ''time out'' kind of activity, something soothing, relaxing, and undemanding.

Not sure what that might be? Use the exercise below to figure out what kinds of milestone celebrations will really please you:

Exercise 2

Check the things you might enjoy doing:

_____ attending an art appreciation class at a museum
_____ joining a walking group
_____ volunteering with a community group
_____ going to a movie of your choice, alone
_____ getting a massage
_____ going to the dentist to get a tooth fixed or bonded
_____ going away for the weekend
_____ spending the day shopping with a friend
_____ getting a professional manicure
_____ going to a rifle, golf, or baseball range
_____ eating lunch or dinner out by yourself in a nice restaurant
_____ going to the theater
_____ going bowling
_____ taking a free two-hour makeup demonstration at a department store
_____ having your hair restyled
_____ renting a boat for an hour—or a day
_____ buying some new tapes or CDs and listening to them
_____ spending the morning alone in a nearby park
_____ setting aside a day to be completely free with no plans
_____ buying tickets to a concert, ballet, or opera
_____ spending an entire day in bed

_____ giving a small party for friends
_____ going on a day-long walking tour with a group and guide
_____ taking a long drive in the country
_____ visiting residents at a local nursing home
_____ visiting a home where you can play with a baby or small child
_____ sitting in on classes at a university
_____ making a date with someone whose conversation you enjoy
_____ taking a totally free day—no errands, work, or obligations
_____ getting a book from the library and spending the day reading it

Now that you've given some thought to what pleases you, begin to plan your next milestone celebration. It will give you something to look forward to and help keep you on the program. You can choose just one activity (or nonactivity) or construct a day—or weekend—celebration by combining several activities.

Next milestone: _____

Celebration: _____

The Ultimate Reward

Rewards are an essential part of the Walk It Off! program. If you, like me, have been used to regarding pleasure as "selfish" or "destructive," it may take some time before you realize how constructive rewarding yourself for exercising can be. When you're in a happy frame of mind, proud of your accomplishments and feeling physically fit and up to the challenges of life, you become a source of positive inspiration for those around you.

External events influence our state of mind, of course, but I've noticed that internal feedback is even more powerful. Sometimes I feel as if there were two voices inside me. One is a relentlessly negative friend, who keeps pointing out what's wrong with my body, career, friends, and family and with the world around me. She talks something like this: "What's the use of going for a walk, or giving yourself a reward? You're never going to look like Miss America; you'll always be short and fighting hard to keep slim; whatever money you make will just get spent anyway; a lot of people have husbands and children a lot better than yours . . ." And on and on and on she talks, tearing me down and criticizing everything around me. Naturally, I don't have to spend very long listening to her before I start feeling discouraged, blue, and totally incapable of doing anything good for myself.

Fortunately, a Sunny Suzanne also lives inside me. She takes a much brighter view of things. "Hey, you might not be Miss America," she says, "But you're looking better at 32 than you ever did before, and you're taking care of your health by walking almost every morning, and you're earning a decent living, and you dearly love your family and are lucky to have them, and they're lucky to have you. And remember what the neighbor told you on Friday—'Just seeing you striding around the reservoir restores my faith.' " After a few minutes of listening to Sunny Suzanne, I'm tying on my sneakers and warming up, raring to go.

The question is, how do we defeat the negative thoughts that pollute our lives and encourage the positive ones that give us motivation and joy?

The secret came to me about two years ago. I came home from work quite exhausted and frustrated by an incident with my bookkeeper that had taken place at the very end of the afternoon. When my husband asked, "How was your day?" I instantly replied: "Just awful." He looked a bit crestfallen, sorry for me, but also, probably, wondering how pleasant I was going to be that evening.

Sorry for being such a downer, I searched for something more positive to say. It took a few minutes for it to surface, but then I said: "Wait a minute, Bart, what am I talking about? My day was not *all* bad. About two o'clock a patient dropped by the office to bring me a present—a five-pound box of lovely chocolates. She told me that she was tremendously grateful for the corrective surgery I had performed: for the first time in ten years she felt no pain in her feet. 'I feel like I'm dancing on air,' she said. 'You're such a wonderful doctor.' "

I gave the chocolates to my secretary to take to the home for the elderly where she volunteers. But I accepted the compliment myself! As I told Bart about this, he perked up, and so did I. I'm fortunate to have work that lets me help other people; it's wonderful to be able to relieve someone's pain. Compared to that, what did a little hassle with my bookkeeper amount to?

Needless to say, Bart and I spent a lovely happy evening together. I realized that I didn't have to be a passive victim of my internal voices. I could control which Suzanne was whispering in my ear, and by keeping my thoughts upbeat, I could share joy, rather than depression, with my family.

So for the last two years, I've taken an active approach to my moods. I find I have much more control than I initially realized over the thoughts that pass through my head. I can tell Negative Suzanne to shut up. I can beckon Sunny Suzanne to take over. I can use my walking time to look at the positive things in my life and rejoice.

The ultimate reward of the Walk It Off! program, then, is to let in the good news about yourself and your life. This is not a simple matter. It takes constant vigilance for me to let good news in. But it's worth it. When you're kind to yourself, it's a lot easier to be kind to everyone else. In order to give effectively, you need to find ways to replenish your energy and your spirits.

Exercise 3

For the last exercise in this chapter, I'd like you to review some of the good things about yourself. Check those that apply to you:

I have good qualities. For example,
_____ I try to be kind to others.
_____ I work hard.
_____ I have a sense of humor.

_____ I try to understand the other person's point of view.
_____ other (be specific) _____

I have important, caring relationships with
_____ spouse
_____ parents
_____ children
_____ grandchildren
_____ friends
_____ colleagues at work
_____ neighbors
_____ other (be specific) _____

I have scored some emotional victories. For example,
_____ I can control my anger.
_____ I'm not as jealous of other people as I once was.
_____ I can tolerate people's differences.
_____ I've learned how to love.
_____ other (be specific) _____

I've gained some control over my need for
_____ junk food
_____ alcohol or drugs
_____ nicotine
_____ pills
_____ other (be specific) _____

I am a success, because
_____ I help support my household.
_____ I am raising a child.
_____ I manage my household affairs.
_____ I have completed my education.
_____ I am progressing in my career.
_____ I have helped purchase material comforts.
_____ I have learned something new recently.

_____ I have begun a walking program.

_____ other (be specific) _____

Note: If you haven't checked at least one item in each of the categories above, go back and redo this exercise when you're in a brighter mood. If you have checked an item in each category, consider what you've said about yourself. Obviously you have:

- good qualities
- important, caring relationships
- emotional victories
- control over your negative habits
- successes at things that are important to you

Not bad. If you quickly review these positive things about yourself while you're warming up for your walk, or as you're nearing the house on your way back, you'll have achieved the ultimate reward: a good mood and a positive self-image!

Habit Building—in a Nutshell

Remember:

- Persistence, not "willpower," is the key to creating a new habit.
- Walk at the same time each day.
- Have a plan for foul weather.
- Reward yourself for each walk with a 15-minute "me break."
- Enter all walks in your Walker's Log.
- Celebrate walking milestones with a major treat.
- Frequently review your three main reasons for walking.
- Reread the "facts" about walking to increase your motivation.

- Ask for help from supportive people and avoid those who discourage you.
- Give yourself some compliments. Remember, you have:

  good qualities
  important, caring relationships
  emotional victories
  control over negative habits
  successes at things that are important to you

- Allow at least 90 days for walking to become a true "habit."

PART

3

ON THE ROAD

"Wow. I'm really doing this!" That was my thought one day, in 1981, after about my fourteenth walk in three weeks. I was amazed that I was actually sticking to this exercise program, even though there were no classes to go to, no outside supervision, no expensive health club dues to be justified. There were still days when I had to drag myself out of the house to walk, but they were getting rarer. More common were days when I tried to prolong the walking experience as long as possible. On nice days, my "me break" was often spent outside, lingering in the park where I had just walked, gazing at the scenery and simply enjoying my peaceful frame of mind.

As I gained confidence that I had finally found a form of exercise I could enjoy and succeed at, I began to consider how to make it even more enjoyable. My first thoughts turned to walking gear: getting a pair of shoes that would let me walk faster and more comfortably, and collecting some accessories and clothing that expressed my new-found interest. Because of the money I'd spent in the past on sports equipment and outfits that I'd never used, I was wary about going on a big shopping trip. But I did spend a long, slow Saturday afternoon selecting just the right walking shoe. And then after yet another few weeks of continuing to walk, I rewarded myself with an afternoon of browsing in a sporting goods store and buying a few inexpensive accessories.

During this period of solidifying my walking habit, I also began to explore a whole range of places to walk. The convenient alternatives turned out to be much wider than I would have dreamed of; they allowed me to negotiate a walk in virtually any weather and find like-minded souls to keep me company.

The chapters in this section are written for the walker who's already in motion. As I said earlier, it's not necessary to wait until you buy the perfect pair of shoes before beginning to walk. But as your commitment to the program grows, you deserve a shoe that will help you along. And while it's not necessary to know all the walking options in your area before getting started, you'll certainly want to consider them once you are started. The chapters in this section will help you make your walking sessions comfortable, safe, varied, and pleasurable.

7

Choosing Shoes for Walking

Your most important item of walking gear is, of course, your shoes. After you've been walking for a week or two, it's time to consider whether you want to buy a special pair. Those comfortable loafers or crepe-soled shoes you might have worn for your first few "walking-readiness" sessions are not ideal for brisk, regular walking. They let the foot slide around too much, inviting injuries. And crepe soles build up heat in the shoe, causing uncomfortable foot perspiration.

Shoes engineered to help the feet hit the ground during running, tennis, aerobic dance, and other sports are not built for walking. Basic sneakers, or Keds, are great for strolling or shopping, but they don't provide the arch support you need for fitness walking.

Walking shoes are really glorified sneakers that have been specially engineered to provide maximum comfort, support, and stability to counteract the unique pressures walking puts on your feet. Today there's a huge selection of walking shoes on the market—more than 200 varieties for just this one activity! It's easy to feel intimidated by the selection, but it actually works in your favor. If you go to a store with a wide selection, you're bound to find a pair with just the right construction, comfort, and fit . . . and even in the color you want!

How much do you need to spend? You'll find some walking shoes that cost as little as $30 and some that soar near the $200 mark. In the long run it pays to spend enough to get a sturdy, well-fitting pair of shoes. The very cheap ones will need to be replaced sooner and may cause an injury. Be prepared to pay about $65 to $70 for a decent pair. If that's a strain on your pocketbook, remember it's often possible to get high-quality shoes on sale. Ask the salesperson when the store usually runs sales. A friend of mine once did that and the next thing she knew the saleswoman had dug up an attractive, well-built pair of last year's model with a tiny price tag.

If you need an unusual width or shoe size, don't believe the salesperson who tells you you'll have to settle for a standard size because "that's all they make." It may be all that particular shoe store stocks, but with a little persistence, you should be able to find walking shoes in all the widths and sizes made for regular shoes. They range from small, narrow women's size 4, quadruple-A, to men's size 17, quadruple-E. If you have trouble locating your size, take out the Yellow Pages and get on the phone. Call around to shoe stores in your area until you locate one that has your size or will order it. That will save you time and frustration.

High heels are bad for your feet, your legs, and your lower back. Every woman knows that. We wear them as an aid to beauty, not health. So it's good to know you burn 10 percent more calories walking in high heels than in flat shoes.

Choose a shoe that's right for the type of walking you plan to do. If you're trekking into the woods for nature walks, you'll need a sturdier shoe with a deeper tread than you will if you're planning on indoor mall-walking. Most important, buy a pair of shoes you think are *attractive*. This advice may sound frivolous, or obvious, but many people fail to heed it. Since enjoyment is a key factor in helping you stick to an exercise program, you don't want walking shoes that make you feel like a clodhopper. Pick shoes that will help you have a good time—that will make you look forward to "stepping out" when you step into them!

Here are some of the other features to look for. A good walking shoe should be:

Sturdy but flexible. The key difference between a walking and a running shoe is that the one for walking must be more flexible over the top of your foot. Your foot bends at a greater angle coming out of each walking step than it does coming out of each running stride, and your shoe should bend with it. Before you try on a shoe, test it with your hands to see if it bends easily around the laces.

Comfortable and roomy. Can you wiggle and stretch your toes? There should be between 1/4 and 1/2 inch of space between your longest toe and the tip of the shoe. A shoe with a squared-off toe area, or "toe box," will give your toes the most room. A sloping toe will put too much pressure on the area. Look for a shoe with a reinforced toe. It will last longer. The reinforcement keeps the toe area from caving in after heavy wear.

Sized for you. You won't necessarily wear the same size in a walking shoe as in your regular shoe wear. If you find that your feet swell during long walks and/or you like to wear heavy socks, consider a shoe a half size larger than you usually wear. When you shop for shoes, take along (or purchase) the socks that you intend to wear and try them on with the shoes. Here's another tip: go shoe shopping late in the afternoon or evening. That's the time of day when your feet are their biggest!

Shoe sizes grow over the years. Constant weight-bearing might cause the feet to spread—especially across the ball of the foot. You may need wider shoes as you age.

Firm at the heel. A firm "heel counter"—a hard plastic cup around the back and lower part of your heel—keeps your heel from shifting around. This helps prevent your ankles from bending inward or outward while you walk, and will help you avoid blisters and injuries. The "heel collar"—the part of the heel counter that surrounds the top of your heel—should be well padded and provide plenty of support. But make sure it's not too stiff or too high for comfort. If the heel collar fits improperly it may hurt the back of your heel and push your ankle into an unnaturally bent-forward position with each step you take.

Padded at the heel. Choose a shoe with plenty of cushioning under the heel and under the ball of the foot. This cushioning is provided by the shoe's "midsole"—the area between the foot bed inside the shoe and the rubber "outsole" on the bottom of the shoe. Cushioning is especially important if you'll be walking on hard surfaces, such as suburban streets or city sidewalks.

Tilted at the toe. The toe of a walking shoe should be slightly raised rather than flat to the ground. The tilted toe helps complete the rocking motion of the natural walking stride.

Raised at the heel. A slightly raised heel is also preferable. It also helps with the rocking of the walking stride. And it reduces the risk of tendon strain. The heel should be about ½ to ¾ inch above the sole of your foot.

Medium-traction. You don't need as much traction in a walking as in a running shoe. The walking shoe's sole should be thinner and its tread less deep than a running shoe's. A heavy tread makes your foot "catch" on the ground with each step. This is useful when you're involved in the faster, more violent action of running; it keeps you from falling or slipping. But it's not as necessary when you walk. A deep tread can cause your foot to "jam" with each step, creating unnecessary resistance. This pushes your toes up against the inside of the front of the shoe, causing discomfort and possible injury.

Cool. The material that forms the upper part of the shoe should not only be sturdy and flexible, but be made of material that "breathes." Some good walking shoes have perforated uppers. This helps the foot stay cool by allowing air to circulate around it as you walk and providing an escape route for perspiration. Canvas and nylon are suitable materials for walking shoes, but if you can spend a little more, leather or leather mesh is probably the ideal. Leather uppers allow the foot to breathe but also provide consistent support. On cold or inclement days, they keep the foot warm and dry.

Soft inside. A padded tongue and an absorbent, smooth inside lining, with no uncomfortable bumps or high seams, is important for comfort and avoiding rubbing and blisters. Run your hand along the inside of the shoe to check the lining.

Relatively lightweight. Walking shoes on the market today range from as little as 4 ounces to more than 16 ounces in weight, depending on the size and style. Heavier shoes do make you work harder with each step and thereby increase the difficulty and aerobic benefit of your routine—but there are better, more gradual ways to increase the difficulty of your walk. Why start out with a burden on your feet?

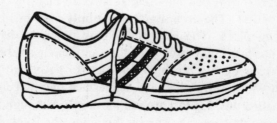

Shopping for Shoes

Try to go shoe shopping on a day when you can spend some time at it. Being in a hurry just adds pressure to what is potentially a pleasant activity. It's also nice if the shoe store is not too crowded when you go in. A salesperson who's willing to take the time to really help you can make the whole experience more satisfying.

Begin by asking the salesperson to show you the selection of walking and running shoes and take a moment to point out the differences in the tread and construction. Once you know which models are for walking, take a close look at each of them. Note differences in price and attractiveness. You may want to try on shoes with quite different styling to see which looks best on your foot. And it's a good idea to try on a very inexpensive and very expensive shoe, even if you don't plan on buying either. This will make you a more educated consumer and help you decide just which features you think are worth paying extra for.

Before trying the shoe on, check for some of the important features: breathability in the upper fabric; a front portion that bends easily; a square toe box and raised heels and toes; a firm heel collar; a layer of padding under the heel and midfoot; a padded tongue and a smooth, seam-free inside lining.

Try to select at least three models that meet these conditions; then, sit down and try them on in your size.

With some shoes, you may realize at once that the construction is wrong for you. The arch may be painfully high or hit your foot in the wrong place. The heel collar may pinch or dig into your ankle. Or the front may give your toes an unpleasant squeeze.

Narrow your choice down to one or two pairs that feel pretty good when you first put them on. Then lace one pair up at a time and give them a walking test around the store. Although I'm willing to let salespeople save me time by threading the laces through the shoes before I try them on, once they're on my foot, I prefer to adjust the tension of the laces myself. It's impossible to tell how a shoe really fits if the laces are too loose or too tight.

I'm never shy about bouncing up and down, jumping, and stretching in the store when I'm trying on shoes. I never decide on a pair until I've answered the following questions:

- Is there room to spread and wiggle the toes?
- Do the heels feel comfortable?
- Are the arches pleasantly supportive?
- Do the shoes rub or create any hot spots?
- Is it the right size?
- Do they feel good on both feet?
- Do they look good?

Usually the final decision about which pair to buy is pretty easy. One pair should make your feet feel so heavenly that you don't even want to take them off to pay for them. If you don't find a pair that gives that level of satisfaction, you may want to try another store. But if you do, noting the brands and models you've already tried and discarded will simplify your second trip.

If you do a good part of your walking on rugged, rocky dirt terrain you may want to buy a second pair of really sturdy hiking shoes. Hiking shoes are heavier than city walking shoes. They have deeper treads and lace high around the ankles to provide stability over rocky surfaces and hills. Many hiking shoes are now built with modern walking-shoe technology, which shortens the breaking-in period and increases comfort. Look for a pair that has the features described for walking shoes.

As you use your new shoes regularly for walking, check them occasionally to make sure the features on the above list are holding up. Is the toe still flexible? The cushioning intact? The tread may get worn down and the support weakened before the outside of the shoe shows much wear and tear. But do replace them once the internal structure is deteriorated to spare yourself the risk of bruises, blisters, and even a twisted ankle.

Walking Shoes in Disguise

One of the great boons of the fitness movement of the past fifteen years is that it helped move the lowly sneaker into the fashion limelight. It wasn't too long ago, remember, that the only comfortable shoes on the market were what Grandma called "sensible shoes"—clunky, laced shoes of heavy leather that signaled that a woman cared more about how her feet felt than how her legs looked.

> *Foot shock* can be caused by wearing shoes that are not properly cushioned when you walk on hard surfaces, such as concrete. Remember, if you weigh 200 pounds, your feet support about 350 to 400 pounds when you walk.

Well, these days Grandma is wearing sneakers, too. And shoe manufacturers have begun to realize that the "sneaker generation" wants a high degree of comfort *and* fashion in all shoes. Fashion historians trace the current style of wearing sneakers with business clothes to a New York City subway strike, when office workers began to walk to work. By the time the strike ended, sneakers with three-piece suits and dresses had become a fashion staple.

I'm one of those women who've held out against this fashion wave. Although I think nylons and walking shoes look rather cute on other women, I don't feel attractive wearing my walking shoes with business clothes. I guess my years of wearing orthopedic shoes as a child have left some permanent scars. So I was particularly thrilled when shoe manufacturers started advertising their new line of "walking pumps."

Walking pumps have a layer of cushioning under the heel and ball of the foot that lessens the impact of each step against the sidewalk. They also have nonslip rubber soles that make walking a pleasure all day long. I now own a selection of these shoes with 1-inch and 1½-inch heels in colors to match my business outfits.

Not only do they take the wince out of walking at work, but they encourage me to sneak in a walk at lunchtime. I still prefer to wear my regular walking shoes for exercise, but these pumps give me more flexibility.

There's also a growing selection of what the shoe industry calls "comfort shoes." On the outside, these shoes look like standard oxfords, loafers, skimmers, wing-tips, moccasins, or hiking boots. But they're engineered inside for walking comfort, and their rubber soles lessen the impact of city streets. Some have special "memory foam" that shapes to your foot to create an individual fit.

As you develop the walking habit, you may find that your feet get "spoiled" by feeling so good in your walking shoes. With the growing selection of more comfortable street shoes, you'll be able to keep them spoiled around the clock.

8

What to Wear in Any Weather

Fog, drizzle, blinding sun, gentle breezes, and whistling winds—the walker meets them all and after a while begins to appreciate the beauty in dank, cloudy weather as well as the perfection of an unexpectedly warm day in January. The key to enjoying all kinds of weather, of course, is dressing for it.

As walking has become a more and more popular form of diversion and exercise, an entire supply industry has sprung up. But it's not necessary to spend a lot of money in order to outfit yourself for walking. All you *really* need is a good pair of walking shoes.

Your closet probably already holds outfits appropriate for walking in most weather. The "comfort" clothes and the spiffier outfit you put together in Chapter 2 will probably serve you for quite a while. The extra things you may need to buy—like earmuffs or insect repellent—will also prove useful when you're not walking.

However, if you can afford it and buying special clothes or equipment adds to your walking pleasure, why not indulge? There are many little pleasures and conveniences on the market that can serve as rewards and incentives to keep up your walking routine. Many people find that putting on their "official" walking outfit is all it takes to get them in the mood to exercise.

Whether you put together a walking outfit at the thrift shop or by mail order from a store based in the Swiss Alps, there are certain qualities you need in your walking clothes:

Breathability. Some fabrics, such as many silks and polyesters, do not "breathe." They're so tightly woven that air doesn't easily pass into the fabric, and perspiration is not absorbed and allowed to escape and evaporate. These fabrics can make you uncomfortably warm as you walk, no matter what the temperature outside. Be sure to avoid clothing made of nonporous fabrics such as rubber or plastic. Yes, I know the advertisements claim they'll make you lose weight. But, in fact, all you lose is water through excess perspiration, and this can be dangerous to your health. Wool, cotton, and cotton-polyester blends are the breathable fabrics that walkers find most comfortable.

Comfort. Underwear that rides up or cuts the thighs, shirts that are tight under the arms, and pants or skirts that bind the waist can make walking a misery. Before you go out for a walk, wiggle and move around in your clothes. If your socks fall down or your clothes pinch the skin, save yourself some misery and change before you go out.

Flexibility. Some clothing that feels fine when you're standing still begins to bind as you swing your arms or flex your hips. Try some pre-walk striding to check.

Protection. Walking should not make any part of your body feel uncomfortable, so if you get sore in places, you need to do something about it. Some men find that wearing a jock strap greatly increases their walking comfort. Women may find their breasts feel uncomfortable during a long walk; a firm sports bra provides support and protection against damage to delicate breast tissue. A sports bra is particularly recommended for women with very large breasts, or those who experience swelling at particular times in the menstrual cycle.

Layering. No matter what the temperature, the amount of clothing you need to feel warm at the beginning of your walk is bound to be too much for the end, when your heart rate and body temperature are up. A T-shirt, a sweater or sweatshirt, and an outer jacket are a good combination for cool weather. As you warm up, you can take off a layer and tie it around your waist.

Hot-Weather Dressing

On truly blistering days, when the temperature is climbing into the 90s and the humidity is high, it may be best to walk indoors—in an air-conditioned shopping mall, gym, or an indoor track. If you want to walk outside, choose the early-morning or evening hours; avoid high noon. Heat prostration and dehydration can be life-threatening, so there's no sense being a hot-weather hero.

However, when the weather is hot but not horrendous, walking can be particularly pleasurable. The whole neighborhood tends to be outside, so walking can be a sociable and interesting activity. There's also a wonderful sense of freedom that comes from getting out sans jackets and scarves. Here are some tips for hot-weather happiness:

Dress as lightly as possible. Track shorts worn with a loose-fitting T-shirt or tank top make a good all-purpose summer walking outfit. If you're a bit shy about exposing that much flesh, loose-fitting cotton pants, like those worn for karate, are a good choice. Women might also consider a long, billowing skirt or culottes.

Choose porous fabrics. Cotton and nylon are the best bets for summer. Rubber or plastic clothing, which I distrust in any weather, is particularly dangerous in summer, when it can cause dehydration, fainting, and heart problems.

Don't skip the socks. Although it may seem cooler to do without them, wearing sneakers without socks can cause chafing. If your feet sweat, they'll feel uncomfortably wet and squishy against the sole of your shoe. Instead, wear thin ankle socks, preferably in cotton to absorb perspiration.

Try a hat. A lightweight, light-colored hat or cap is handy for keeping the sun off your head. If it has a brim, it will also shade your face. On the hottest day, some walkers like to dip their caps in cold water before they leave to keep their heads cool throughout the walk.

Some prefer visors. A sun visor won't protect your scalp from the sun's rays, but it will keep the sun off your face. Some people find visors more comfortable than hats.

Always wear sunscreen. If possible, apply sunscreen to your face and all exposed skin about 30 minutes before you go out. This gives it a chance to penetrate your skin. Fair-skinned people need a sunscreen with a protection factor of 15 or higher. Experiment with different brands until you find one that smells pleasant and applies easily.

Consider portable sunscreen. If you take long walks and want to reapply sunscreen, you can buy a flexible bracelet full of sunscreen, and squeeze it on as you walk. These bracelets are popular with teenagers at the beach and are often sold in the junior beachware departments or at boardwalk stores.

Moisturizers are an option. Moisturizers can reduce the effectiveness of sunscreens, so don't load them on before you go out. But do apply them when you come back from your walk to keep your skin in good condition.

Don't forget the sunglasses. Tinted glasses protect your eyes from the harsh rays of the sun and help you see where you're going. Under a new federal law, sunglasses must now carry a label that tells you how much protection they give you against damaging sunlight and which outdoor activities they're appropriate for.

Consider insect repellent. If your walking route takes you through wooded areas or tall grass, and especially if you live in an area where there's a danger of Lyme disease, it's advisable to apply insect repellent before you leave the house. It is available in lotion, liquid, and spray forms, and in small containers that can be tucked in a pocket for reapplication.

Take along some water. Some walkers can plan their route to go by a public water fountain. Otherwise, it's a good idea to carry some with you when the temperature is 80 degrees or above. Drink about 2 ounces of water before you leave the house, and take along 3 to 6 ounces for every 20 minutes you plan to walk.

Use water bottles as hand weights. Two plastic bottles of water can serve the double purpose of handweights and a water supply. Or you may want to invest in a water bottle that can be clipped to your belt, or in a spray bottle like those that professional football players use to squirt water into the mouth. On the very hottest days, you can cool off by washing your face or pouring some water over your head.

Cold-Weather Dressing

Is it 5 degrees below zero with high winds and ice on the ground? Don't be a hero. Find a place to walk indoors. There's a limit to just how "invigorated" you should feel from exercising in below-freezing temperatures.

But being sensible doesn't mean you should shy away from walking on a sunny 25-degree day. A brisk winter walk can make you feel wonderfully healthy and virtuous. I began my walking program in the winter and have developed a special affection for winter walking. Still, I don't enjoy feeling chilled to the bone. I want to feel just as comfortable walking on a frigid day as on a warm one, so I pay careful attention to what I wear.

> The English Romantic poet William Wordsworth is said to have walked 14 miles a day for a total of 180,000 miles in his lifetime.

Think insulation. In cold weather you need to construct your own personal heating system that uses the heat your body generates as it walks. Layers of clothing act as barriers to the cold, very much like insulation in a house or apartment. Warm air is trapped in between the layers and held next to your body. The more you walk, the warmer the air becomes. So remember, the combination of a long-sleeved shirt and a medium-weight sweater is warmer than just one very bulky sweater.

Don't skimp on clothing. Always overdress, rather than underdress, for cold weather. If you begin to feel too warm after walking for a few minutes, you can always peel off a layer and tie the extra clothing around your waist.

Long underwear can be a luxury. If you've never worn long underwear, you're in for a treat. The warmth and comfort it provides can change you from a winter hater to a winter lover. Inexpensive cotton long johns are a good investment; you'll find yourself wearing them for winter walks and other occasions. For a treat, consider the new luxury underwear available in department stores. Paper-thin silk and cotton knits have a luxurious lingerie look, but the most luxurious thing is the warmth they provide.

Choose toasty fabrics. Your inner layer of clothing should be made of a material that absorbs perspiration, such as fine wool, silk knits, or cotton. The middle layer should be a warm material, perhaps knitted wool or synthetic pile. The outer layer should be made of a material that repels water and also "breathes," allowing some perspiration to escape so that you don't feel drenched in your own sweat. The type of fabric in windbreakers is ideal. Most winter outerwear comes in dark colors—navy, black, brown—for a good reason: dark colors absorb and retain heat from the sun and will make you feel toasty on the chilliest days.

Hats are in. Your mother was right: most of your body heat escapes through your head in the winter. So wear a warm hat or cap. Earmuffs are a delightful accessory. And owning a pair gives you more flexibility in choosing a hat; you don't have to search for one that covers your ears. For women, a wool scarf and earmuffs can substitute for a hat.

Scarves are a must. Many people forget that the neck is also an exposed part of the body. If you're comfortable in turtlenecks, a lightweight one is good neck protection. But there's nothing like a soft wool scarf for keeping your neck toasty. And you can pull it up to protect your chin and mouth if a cold wind starts blowing.

Choose smart socks. It's crucial to keep your feet warm and dry during winter walks. Heavy cotton or wool socks, warm and absorbent, are a must. You might try wearing two pairs of socks at the same time—but only if your shoes are roomy enough to accommodate them without constricting or rubbing your feet and toes.

Consider a ski mask. A pull-down mask is a good friend on windy winter days, or when temperatures get into the teens. When the wind is in your face, it protects your skin against frostbite; when the wind is at your back and the sun feels warm, simply pull up the mask and enjoy the warm rays.

Keep your fingers warm. In very cold weather, use mittens rather than gloves. Mittens keep the fingers and palm together, creating a nice warm airspace. If you don't own mittens, try using a pair of woolen socks.

Protect your skin. Skiers know that the winter sun can do almost as much skin damage as the summer rays. Wear sunscreen on all exposed skin. And wear sunglasses, especially when harsh rays are reflected by snow and ice. Mirrored sunglasses give extra protection against this kind of reflected glare. To protect your skin from chapping, coat your lips and face lightly with Vaseline.

Put it all together. Here's a possible outfit for when the temperature outside is, say, 15 degrees and windy: warm underwear, top and bottom; a thin turtleneck shirt and tights or a pajama bottom; a sweater and a pair of wool pants; a jacket of tightly woven fabric; a pair of cotton socks covered by a pair of wool ones; scarf, hat, face mask, and mittens.

Wet-Weather Dressing

You've heard of people who "don't know enough to come in out of the rain." Well, I'm one of them. I don't go out to walk in a downpour or a thunderstorm. But a walk in drizzly, warm rain or a soft, powdery snowfall gives me a tremendously light-hearted, free, childlike feeling.

Here's how to dress for a walk in the rain:

Wear a rain cloak. A jacket-length or, even better, full-length parka is the ideal rain gear. The best are made out of breathable waterproof material such as Gore-tex, Entrant, Ultrex, or Thin-tech. Look for one with a minimum number of seams and pockets—even waterproof seams may leak. Some rain gear now comes with Velcro wrist and pocket seals. If you can't find a suitable parka in a department store, try a sporting goods or camping store. Such stores usually have a good selection of reasonably priced rain gear. Try to get a parka that's roomy enough to fit over your winter jacket so you can wear it in all seasons.

Search for a rain hat. A good, wide-brimmed, waterproof rain hat with a strap under the chin to keep it from flying off in the rain is one of my proudest possessions. It took me several years to find one that didn't make me look like the Wicked Witch of the West, but I finally found a flattering style in a camping gear store. I prefer to use a hat rather than the hood on my parka. Most hoods block your vision when you turn to the side, and they tend to let the rain run down your face.

Boots are an option. If you can find a waterproof boot that's truly comfortable, fine. But most of the rubber ones I've tried make my feet too hot during a long walk. If you have leather walking shoes, they'll probably stay leakproof unless you're in a really heavy downpour or you step in a puddle. Use waterproofing sprays on occasion to create a better seal.

Take an umbrella if you must. I'm not wild about walking with an umbrella because I can't swing my arms. But if the only chance I have to walk is on my way to business, I have no choice unless I want to arrive looking like a drowned rat. I like to use a long, wide umbrella with a wooden handle. Then if the rain stops I can use it as a walking stick.

Although I've been walking for almost a decade now, I must say that I'm still wearing many of the walking clothes I bought during my first year. It sounds silly, but I've developed a special affection for my track shorts, my rabbit earmuffs, my favorite walking shoes, and my shiny blue rain hat that took so long to find. These clothes have become part of the very personal pleasure I take in walking.

So now that your commitment to walking is growing, be sure to reward yourself now and again with items of clothing that increase your comfort and your pleasure. You deserve it!

What to Take Along

Most of the time you'll need to carry some things with you when you're off for your walk. For safety's sake, always have some kind of identification on you. I leave a business card inside the pocket of the jacket I wear for walking. You may need a medical alert tag that lists any health problems and allergies, or an ''I wear contacts'' tag.

I also carry change for the telephone just in case I run into trouble and need to call home. Usually, you'll also need to bring along your housekeys, and perhaps sunglasses and a watch. Your jacket or sweatshirt pocket may be sufficient for stashing these items, but if that makes you feel bulging and overloaded, consider buying some sort of carrying pack that leaves your arms free.

Here are some of the items easily found in sporting goods, camping, and even some sports shoe stores that can add to your walking pleasure.

Water Bottles

These come in all shapes and sizes, from the traditional canteen with a shoulder strap to newfangled plastic bottles that clip on your belt. And, as I mentioned earlier, a plastic bottle of mineral water in each hand serves the double purpose of a water supply and hand weight.

Carrying Pack

One item I recommend you consider buying is a backpack or a waistpack—more commonly called a "fanny pack." These give you an easy way to carry things you want to bring along on your walk without interfering with your arm swinging. They also store very useful pieces of clothing—scarf, gloves, outer jacket—you no longer want to wear once you warm up. If you walk in the woods, a pack really comes in handy. You can carry bug repellent, sunscreen, water, maps, healthy snacks, and even a book to read when you're ready for a rest.

And owning a pack may encourage you to walk more. For example, you can walk to the post office, carrying your packages, or walk to do your errands and have an easy way to carry home purchases.

Pedometer

A pedometer—a small, lightweight mileage counter—is a popular walking "extra." It attaches to your shoe or your waist, and helps you keep track of how far you've gone. A pedometer is especially helpful if you regularly vary your walking routes or are gradually increasing the distance you walk. It helps keep you honest and increases your sense of accomplishment.

Notebook and Pencil

If you're like me, you'll have some of your most brilliant thoughts while you're walking. Suddenly, the answer to a pressing problem at work, or in dealing with your children, will occur to you. I like to be able to write it down on the spot and get on to thinking about other things. If I don't have a pad and pencil with me, I get nervous that I'll forget my insight and so I keep rerunning it in my head.

Some people like to carry their Walker's Log with them and make notes as they go, rather than recording when they get home as I do. You can use a regular variety-store notebook for this, or buy a special "exercise log" with daily entries to complete. These are now sold in many sporting goods stores and bookstores.

Walking Sticks

Walking sticks are a good way to prevent falls, says Dr. Robert Sleight, director of the Walking Association in Arlington, Virginia: "A wooden one bought in a store, or even a straight, sturdy branch, would do just fine. A staff can be used to give extra support and balance, and is good exercise for the arms."

Walking sticks have been a collectible for many years now, and some antique shops have a fascinating selection. Some modern walking sticks even have seats that fold out for an impromptu rest.

The Walkman Question

Should you wear a stereo headset when you walk? Many walkers I know use them to listen to music, inspirational or instructional tapes, books-on-tape, or one of the many walking audiotapes recorded specifically for walkers.

I myself am wary of using a headset when I walk. I find it blocks my hearing and makes me miss much of what's going on around me. I prefer to stay alert to the sounds of passing traffic, other walkers or runners, bicyclists, and slippery ground surfaces.

If you walk on an outdoor or indoor track in a safe area, using a headset is probably safe. But be careful about enveloping yourself in sound when you're out on city sidewalks or suburban streets.

Walking Tapes

Some beginning walkers find that listening to audiotapes about walking as they walk helps them keep going. They're available in bookstores, sporting goods stores, record stores, and some department stores. Magazines written for walkers and other fitness enthusiasts also carry ads for mail-order sources of tapes. Prices range from about $6 to $20.

Most of these tapes include:

- instructions for warm-up and cool-down exercises
- instructions for particular walking and breathing techniques
- music (some tapes have music with a strong beat; others have different selections with increasing tempos)
- encouragement (this may be especially helpful for people who can't find a partner or walking group and need some outside motivation)
- discussions of the various exercise benefits of walking
- supplemental information booklets

Also available are a number of walking videotapes, sold in video and other retail stores, that show as well as tell you about the best way to walk. The problem, of course, is that you can't take them with you as you walk. So you need to remember the advice and try it out later, rather than directly following the instructions given on an audiotape during your walking routine. Videos cost about $20 to $50 a tape.

Insect Repellent

Nothing's guaranteed to spoil a walk as much as a swarm of black flies or mosquitoes that travel along with you. And in some areas, ticks have become a real health threat because they carry Lyme disease, a hard-to-diagnose, dangerous illness. When you go out for warm-weather walks, avoid wearing hair spray, after-shave lotion, or perfumed cosmetics. These smells attract bugs.

Commercially available insect lotions and sprays are a good idea if you're walking in a buggy area. A bee-sting and medical kit are necessary if your walk takes you far from civilization. In the woods, long pants, socks, and a long-sleeved shirt are essential for protecting against ticks. Rangers recommend that you wear light colors—tan or white. These attract fewer bugs and also make it possible for you to notice and remove any ticks that may have adhered to your clothing.

9

Where to Walk Safely

If you did the walking-readiness exercises in Chapter 2, you've already given at least some cursory attention to the walking routes available near your home or workplace. In this chapter, I encourage you to stretch your imagination. Become a tourist in your own neighborhood and view its points of interest as if for the first time. No matter where you live, I bet there are unexplored nooks and crannies that offer opportunities for interesting walks—a small nature reserve, an old cemetery, a park with a waterfall.

There are probably also interesting places that are nearby, but too far to walk to. On days that you have some extra time, you can drive a car to get there and then walk. Other places might make a long and interesting one-way walk, from which you'll hop on a bus to return.

Some of my very favorite walks have a treat at the end. On occasion, I walk up to a university area about 2 miles from my house, then take a rest browsing through a used-book shop. I usually return with a book in each hand serving as handweights. On Sundays, my family and I sometimes walk about 1½ miles to a brunch place we like, and then stroll back. It's not a real workout for me, but I figure it's better than *driving* to the brunch place and it sets a good example for the children.

This chapter will give you some ideas about how to find the best surfaces for walking, where to get information about walking trails and tracks, how to cope with city sidewalks, and—very important—how to enhance your safety when walking in various settings. But its main purpose is to inspire you to get out and explore your own neighborhood and find those delightful, hidden places that are accessible only on foot.

The Search for Springy Surfaces

A smooth, warm sand beach is my first choice for a walking surface. I have to watch out for sharp stones, shells, and perhaps jellyfish, but that's a small price to pay for the pleasurable workout the sand gives to the muscles in my bare feet (not to mention the wonderful view of the ocean). If I'm at the beach on a cool day, I usually keep my walking shoes *on* and walk at the edge of the beach far from the water, where the sand is not soft as it is close to the water. Walking on sand or dirt takes a lot more energy and burns more calories than walking on a harder surface. So on my first day of a beach vacation, I cut back a bit on my walking speed, or the total time out, to avoid achy calves the next day.

If I can't have the beach, my second choice is to walk on a packed-dirt or rubberized-asphalt surface. A path in the woods or across a park is wonderful when available. I try to avoid walking on deep, loose dirt or clumpy grass. It's hard to get good traction on these surfaces, but easy to turn an ankle, stumble, or fall.

Walking on sand or dirt can boost your energy expenditure by as much as a third. It also exercises more of the muscles in the foot, especially if you walk barefoot.

Most often I end up at the location nearest my home—the springy surface of a smooth outdoor path around the reservoir in Central Park. The packed-dirt surface is easy to manage, so I can walk at my fastest. Some people complain that going around and around a circular path or track gets boring. I seldom find it so. Since I don't have to worry about traffic or directions, I can let my thoughts and fantasies soar freely and my laps are over before I know it.

The rubberized asphalt on indoor tracks in health clubs and high schools also provides good traction, safety, and a springy surface. One tip: if the track is slanted, be sure to walk clockwise one day and counterclockwise the next. Otherwise you'll overuse one leg and underuse the other.

Suburban streets and city sidewalks present hard concrete or asphalt surfaces. Indoor malls and office buildings also have hard walking surfaces; some may be slippery because they've recently been washed and waxed. All of these can be hard on the feet unless your walking shoes are well cushioned. But with the right pair of shoes, these most convenient and available surfaces will do quite nicely.

Sidewalk Savvy

Many of my walks are on city streets. I try to plan my routes so I don't have to stop often for streetlights or traffic obstructions. I usually weave my way along the side streets of Manhattan rather than try to maneuver along the avenues, which are more heavily traveled and have much shorter blocks. One great plus about walking on city sidewalks is that it's usually relatively easy to keep track of your mileage. In New York, we estimate that a mile equals twenty north-south city blocks.

The best thing about city walks is how interesting they can be. I've explored some old residential neighborhoods with beautiful houses and historic buildings. I've walked past the most expensive shops in the world. I've traveled through neighborhoods where so little English is spoken that I could be in another country. My technique for making sure the sights don't distract me from getting a workout is to keep up a brisk pace for 30 minutes, noting the places I'd like to stop and look at longer. Then I take the same route back and allow myself to stop now and then and satisfy my curiosity.

Walking in the city is seldom totally relaxing. It's necessary to stay alert and aware of all kinds of possible dangers. Some walkers I know wear a safety whistle around their necks with the hope that the shrill sound, known to police, will attract help if there's a problem.

I don't hesitate to cross the street to avoid passing people who look dangerous or unfriendly, or duck into the nearest store if I suspect someone might be following me. And, in general, I try to keep away from uninhabited places. If I'm thinking of exploring a new route, I do it with friends, or in a car, first, to make sure it meets my safety needs. When I'm in a strange city on business, I always ask the hotel clerk to recommend a safe place to walk. Unfortunately, there are few areas in few cities where I feel comfortable walking alone at night.

Cars are another danger in a big city. One of the hardest things for me is to force myself to wait for the light to change, instead of dodging the traffic. The standard recommendation is to walk in place until the light turns green to keep your heart rate up. I admit, I usually feel too self-conscious to do this, though I encourage more confident readers to give it a try.

Find the Green

Wherever you live, it's probably possible to find a green grassy area, away from motor traffic, to walk in. Most cities and towns have lots of parks, and even a small one will do, if you don't mind circling it a number of times. The perimeter of a golf club, a college campus, or a landscaped industrial park might be suitable.

> *Walking up a mild, 14-degree slope* requires four times the effort of walking on level ground. Going downhill requires more energy, too! The braking you do when going down a slope uses more muscle power than walking on a straight, flat surface.

One reason I walk so often in Central Park is that it gets me away from car fumes and traffic noise. The scenery there is prettier and more relaxing than the streets. The park also has lots of hills and staircases that I use to increase the challenge of my exercise.

The drawbacks of parks and other green areas is that they may be deserted and dangerous at times. The best protection is the old saw "There's safety in numbers." Try to find a friend or two, or a whole club, to walk with you. Walk at times when the park is full of mothers with small children. If you're walking alone and you see another walker, take a risk and ask if you can buddy up for safety. You don't have to get into a big conversation. Just travel together to keep each of you from looking like an easy crime victim.

Suburban and Country Roads

Of the 50,000 people a year killed in automobile accidents, 10,000 are pedestrians. Hazards from cars are especially hard to avoid in the suburbs and country, where there are often no sidewalks. It's best to choose wide, noncurvy roads for your walk. Walk facing the oncoming traffic and avoid walking at dusk, at night, and in fog when visibility is poor.

If you're a suburban walker, try to vary the time of day and your route when you walk. A strict, reliable routine makes it easy for burglars, watching the house, to figure out when you're gone.

Hiking over rough paths and terrain burns up to 50 percent more calories than walking on smooth, level ground. So hit those trails when the weather's right.

Unleashed dogs are another scourge of walkers. The standard advice is not to look scared (a rigid body, a pained face) if a dog approaches; in fact, pretend you're not looking at it at all. If the dog seems about to charge, shout "Down!" If it does attack, hit it in the snout with your arm, or a stick or stone. Another approach is to carry a walking stick for ready protection, or buy a can of dog-away spray at a pet shop. But I think the most practical tactic is to try to avoid these encounters to begin with by getting to know where the dogs in the neighborhood live and making a wide circle around their turf. You can take a dog-watching tour in your car first to check out the territory.

In the country, narrow rural roads can be hazardous. Watch out for ditches and fast-approaching vehicles. In fields and hilly areas, keep your eye out for holes, tree stumps, and other obstacles.

Good places to walk include paths that border rivers and streams or encircle ponds and lakes. These make pleasant walking routes when they're not too muddy or slippery.

"I have never jogged or run because I can't see the flowers, shrubs, and trees. My form of madness is strolling, and preferably up hills with views and flora."—WILLIAM DOCK, M.D., professor of medicine

To find the best tracks and paths in suburban and country areas you may have to drive to your walk. Check out the local high school, community center, or recreation department. Also, ask longtime local residents about nature preserves and trails in your area. It's amazing what wonderful paths can be right under your nose, but out of sight unless you know how to find them.

Tips for Night Walkers

During the winter months when it gets dark early, walking in the early morning or at lunchtime is a good alternative. By the time most of us come home at night, it's already dark outside. If you do choose to walk at night, try to enroll a walking buddy to come with you. Or walk in well-lit, populated areas.

> "I walk half the daylight, but when I tell people, I don't think they believe me."—HENRY DAVID THOREAU

Wearing white at night is a good idea. Reflective material sewn on your outerwear and wrapped on walking stick and reflective tape on the soles of your shoes are recommended. The lights of oncoming cars will bounce off the reflective material and enable the driver to see you. In areas without streetlights, carrying a small flashlight is essential. Stay away from unlit paths, isolated roads, and other areas where you may be vulnerable to assault.

Mall Walking

Don't scoff. Where else can you find miles of smooth corridor and staircases that are safe from rain, snow, blistering heat, broken sidewalks, automobile fumes, dangerous dogs, and dangerous people?

If you're picturing yourself trying to walk briskly in a mall full of Christmas shoppers, think again. Quite a number of malls now open their doors to walkers at 7:00 or 8:00 a.m., long before the stores are open and the shoppers arrive. Some store owners even offer walkers free orange juice, coffee, and rolls, drawings for prizes, and discounts on footwear, shoes, T-shirts, sweat suits, health food, and cosmetics. Walking clubs get to meet around the tables in the cafeteria. And some coordinate with local hospitals to sponsor free blood-pressure and cholesterol testing and arrange for medical specialists to talk at club meetings.

The Walk for Wellness club at the Georgia Square mall near Athens, Georgia, began in 1985 and has over 200 participants who meet monthly. On any given day, twenty-five to forty members will be walking before store hours, some in groups, some in couples or singly. The mall has a bulletin board where walkers update their total walking mileages. Most of the walkers at Georgia Square are aged 55 to 70, with about six women for every four men. But on weekends and holidays this group is joined by teenagers.

Even if mall walking is not for you as a regular routine, you should make a few calls and find out about the hours you can walk at nearby shopping centers. Then you have a ready alternative when a two-week heat wave or cold or rainy spell makes outdoor walking impossible. If the mall has two or more levels, you can get extra exercise (and more complete window shopping) by changing levels with each circuit.

Safety tip for mall walking: Don't put your car in the far corner of the parking lot and exercise by walking across. Instead, park at Saks and walk *through* the mall to get to Macy's.

Health Clubs and Indoor Tracks

Indoor tracks, treadmills, and stair-climbing machines are a great substitute for an outdoor walk when the weather is inclement. Before you plunk down your money for an expensive health club, check out the schools in your area. Many of them are underpopulated these days and offer their gym facilities to local residents at a small cost.

If you do decide to join a health club, be sure to visit it during the hours you intend to use it. A friend of mine signed up in a nearly empty club at 10:00 a.m. on a day off, only to find it unpleasantly packed at 6:00 p.m. when he wanted to use it.

Walking at 3 miles per hour requires the same energy as bicycling at 5 mph. If you walk at 4 mph you're burning as much energy as a cyclist doing 10 mph.

Indoor tracks are usually smaller than outdoor tracks, and you may have to go around dozens of times to complete your walk. This is one place it's quite safe to use a portable radio or tape recorder with earphones, if that helps cut the boredom. You can also walk with a friend, or give yourself some thinking work to do as you walk.

Treadmills are conveyer belts that provide a kind of "track" in a small space. The motorized version allows you to set the speed, and then forces you to walk at it. Some can be elevated at one end to make you walk uphill and increase the exercise challenge.

On nonmotorized treadmills, your legs do all the work and you determine the speed. But the machines can usually be adjusted to allow greater or lower resistance. If your feet get hot after some time on a nonmotorized treadmill, you may be too fast a walker to use this type of machine comfortably.

Walking in Water

And now for something completely different. Don't worry, I won't insist that you walk *on* water. But why not *in* water? It may sound silly, but try it before you laugh. It can be one of the most challenging, relaxing, and rewarding ways to use walking as an exercise.

You can get a good workout by walking through knee- or thigh-deep water along the edge of a lake, stream, or ocean—or by doing walking "laps" in the shallow end of a swimming pool. Walking in water is double exercise because your legs are pushing against water. The payoff for this extra work: you'll burn about 460 calories per hour of water-walking, rather than the 225 or so you burn on flat, dry ground.

But despite the fact that it's harder, many people don't feel any extra strain. In fact, the water has such a soothing, pampering, bathing effect on their bodies that they don't feel they're exercising at all.

If you want to give this a try, take these precautions:

- Remember that no matter how picturesque the setting or how lovely the water feels, you are working your muscles. So you still need to do warm-up stretching.
- Start out in very shallow—ankle- or calf-deep—water. This makes for a lot of splashing, but walking in mid-thigh-deep water is too difficult for beginners.
- Walk more slowly than you do on land. Don't knock yourself out trying to keep up a "pace." Just enjoy the activity and move as fast as you can comfortably and safely.
- Wear shoes! Even the bottom of a pool can make your feet feel rough and sore. And the shallow water along a lake or ocean can conceal sharp rocks, broken glass, and slimy vegetation. Lightweight canvas sneakers will do fine. Some athletic-shoe manufacturers are now making "water shoes."

Recreational Walks

As you build up strength, walking long distances for long hours will become easier and easier for you. That means you'll get greater enjoyment out of recreational activities that require a lot of walking. A trip to one of the following places is a great reward for sticking to your walking program:

- amusement park
- arboretum
- botanical garden

- city neighborhood
- wildlife preserve or forest
- canal towpath or railroad bed
- long bridge
- national or state park
- museum
- historical site
- zoo
- guided nature or city walk

If you don't have ready companions to accompany you on such trips, check with the local Y, library, church or temple, or parks and recreation department for special-interest clubs. Or contact one of the walking clubs in your area. Whether you're interested in nature, art, history, or just chatting, there's bound to be a local group. Some communities have walking groups geared for moms who push strollers! Even if the club doesn't turn out to be your cup of tea, it's a good place to meet a walking companion.

PART

4

THE WALKER'S DIET

If losing weight is your main motivation for walking, you may turn to this section first. Read on, if you're curious, but I strongly encourage you to attain a firm walking habit *before* you attempt to drastically alter your diet. The walking habit will help give you the strength, determination, and upbeat mood you'll need to conquer the unhealthy eating practices you may have developed over the years.

If losing weight is *not* your goal, I encourage you to read this section anyway. For healthy eating involves more than weight control. Study after study has shown that the low-fat, high-on-the-vegetables, rice and pasta diet that's encouraged in these chapters is the best ammunition we have for preventing chronic diseases.

> *One advantage to being overweight*: you burn more calories for every step you take. A 125-pound woman burns 66 calories a mile, walking at 3 miles per hour. Her 175-pound friend burns 92 calories for the same distance and speed.

The principles in the Walker's Diet will be familiar to anyone who has read the preceding chapters. Happy eating, like happy walking, is the goal. I have found, through long and miserable experience, that a punishing, depriving diet simply does not work. Instead, we need to harness our natural urge toward pleasure to an eating plan that is good for body and soul, and keeps us in a good mood!

10

The Happy Eater

Before I became a walker, I was a diet junkie. There was no diet idea too wild, too absurd, or too expensive for me to try. The drinking man's diet of steak and martinis? Sounded good! The grapefruit-and-celery diet? I was game! Liquid meal substitutes? Diet centers that charged $14 a day for food that tasted like cardboard? I believed! All you had to do was promise that I was going to lose 14 pounds in 14 days and I signed on the dotted line.

I can joke about it now, but all those crazy diet attempts were not funny at the time. I weighed 178 pounds after the birth of my second daughter in 1981. I was desperate to lose weight. I was so obsessed with feeling fat that it interfered with my enjoyment of everything. I was uncomfortable going out for an evening with my husband, giving a talk to doctors at my hospital, even meeting my older daughter's nursery school teacher. I was so self-conscious about how I looked that I assumed everyone else was judging me by my dress size.

Well, it won't surprise you that eating steak, grapefruit, liquid meals, and diet-center dinners did not turn me model-thin. Neither did the glitzier, more expensive methods I tried. I visited fat farms for "vacations." (Yes, it's true: there's a black market in potato chips, salami, and beer at those places. I capped the tiny low-calorie dinners with illegal midnight snacks.) My most dangerous dieting experiment, however, was at the hands of a medical doctor who gave mysterious "shots." The shots had a miraculous effect on my appetite: it disappeared. I wasn't hungry, ever. I was very excited! Surely this diet was going to work. The very thought of food turned my stomach.

Can you pinch more than an inch around your hips? Every 1/4 inch over an inch you can grasp from your love handles equals 10 pounds of fat.

Unfortunately, within a week I realized that the "miracle appetite suppressant" had some very unpleasant side effects. I felt "wired" all the time, I alienated everyone I knew with my suddenly hot temper and irritability, and it took hours for me to fall asleep at night. The "miracle drug" was, of course, an amphetamine. Fortunately for my health, and my marriage, I gave it up before I became addicted. And "Doctor Feelgood" has since been stripped of his license.

That experience had a sobering effect on me. I realized I had a very serious need to lose weight and that I needed to address it in a serious way. I knew I *could* lose weight. Each of those crazy diets had "worked," in their way. I'd drop 10, or even 20 pounds until I was triumphantly "finished" with the diet. Then I'd gain the weight back so quickly that my old oversized clothes were still handy in the closet.

But finally I got smart. I swore off "quickie" diets, and at the same time swore off rowing machines, racquetball, running, and other exercises I hated. I began my walking program, and decided to wait until I had done it consistently for six weeks before making a serious attempt to lose weight.

The walking program helped cut down some of my craving for food. Instead of turning to the refrigerator when I felt tired and out of sorts, I went for a walk. By the time I came back my appetite had normalized. A poached apple satisfied me; I didn't need half a dozen doughnuts.

> *If you diet without exercising,* about one-third of the weight you lose is from lean tissue, not fat tissue. This can lead to weakness and muscle wasting.

Between the calories burned by walking and the cutting back on food binges, I lost 5 pounds during my first six weeks of walking. Those 5 pounds meant more to me than the dozens I'd lost and gained through slapdash methods. I rewarded myself by having a few dresses altered to fit my slightly slimmer shape. I had my hair restyled. And I carefully and consciously built up the confidence I needed to try a more organized weight-loss program.

I also began to do some research on what science can actually tell us about good ways to lose weight. Out of this I devised an eating plan for myself based on the principles of good nutrition *and* the foods I enjoyed preparing and eating. Sticking to this plan and continuing to walk four or five times a week helped me lose 58 pounds, slowly, over the course of a year and a half. And those are 58 pounds I haven't had to look at again for the past nine years.

The Happy Eater plan that you're about to read about developed out of my own weight-loss experience and that of my friends and colleagues. It's as suitable for those readers who are *not* overweight as it is for those who are. The food plan incorporates all the latest scientific knowledge about how nutrition affects our immediate mood and energy levels and our long-range chances of getting heart disease, certain forms of cancer, and osteoporosis. It will help you maintain the weight that's right for your body and give you added energy that will help you stick to the Walk It Off! program.

In one sense, the Happy Eater food plan is a conventional diet:

it helps you consciously alter your food intake so that you lose weight. But it doesn't involve the misery, pain, self-deprivation, or great feats of self-control or willpower we usually associate with dieting. And it isn't a conventional diet—that is, it isn't a brief period of unnatural eating after which you return, gratefully, to your old food habits.

Instead, the Happy Eater plan builds on what you've learned about forming new habits in the previous chapters. It includes both the facts and the feelings we have about what we eat and encourages you to express your own individuality and create an eating plan that you can stick to because you like it!

> *Walking and running burn* about the same number of calories *per mile,* though it takes almost twice as long to cover the mile when you're walking. Briskly walking 1 mile in 15 minutes uses the same number of calories as jogging an equal distance in 8½ minutes.

So even if you have a long history of diet failures and have broken every vow you've ever made to yourself about dieting, this is one plan you can succeed with. It's gradual, it's slow, it's easy, and it's also failure-proof. That's because it reviews certain basic facts about healthy eating, puts you in touch with your personal food preferences and problems, and then lets you develop your diet plan based on the foods that you enjoy.

The Facts

Why do we eat more than we need to survive? In a fascinating study by scientists at the University of Chicago, large groups of people were given beepers to carry around with them. When the beepers went off, at random times during the day, they wrote down what they were doing and rated their mood. The results are enough to make any potential dieter giggle. People of all ages and occupations reported that they were happiest during the same single activity: eating.

To me this study, more than any other, explains why so many diets fail. If what you eat makes you feel unhappy—or even neutral—you're killing one of life's more reliable sources of pleasure. So the one immutable rule in the Happy Eater food plan is that for each meal you must choose something you will *enjoy* eating.

"Ha!" you may be thinking. "This diet plan had better include chocolate eclairs and french-fried potatoes." Well, it doesn't, of course. My premise is that with a little self-examination and experimentation you can find dishes you truly enjoy made from the very broad range of foods that are healthy and can help you lose weight.

To lose 1 pound a week you need to use up 3,500 calories more a week than you take in. Walking (3 miles for 5 days) will burn up about 1,500 calories. You then have to shave only 200–400 calories a day from your food intake to achieve your goal.

Before we consider what foods and dishes are going to make dieting work for you, it helps to know a little something about the health-giving and health-robbing properties of food and how they fill your body's nutritional needs. Here's a brief rundown of the basic dietary substances and how they work.

Protein: A Little Bit Will Do You

Proteins are the building blocks of life. All cells in our bodies contain proteins, and they're essential components of muscle, bones, skin, and blood. Proteins allow us to grow, heal, repair old tissue, and transport nutrients to all cells in the body. Proteins are also an important part of our immune system.

The body cannot store protein; it must be provided daily through our diet. However, as a society, Americans consume too much protein. Our dinners are often built around a 12-ounce steak or a Sunday roast. And while some protein is essential, too much is bad for your health. The body does not use excess protein; it stores it as fat.

The most popular sources of protein—meats and dairy products—are laden with saturated fats and calories. Eating too much animal protein can lead to clogged arteries and heart disease. Vegetable proteins, such as dried beans, grains, nuts and seeds, provide better proteins without the dangerous fats. There have been countless studies showing that people who consume legumes and vegetables have fewer clogged arteries than those who eat diets rich in animal proteins. Too much protein can rob calcium from our bones, which leads to bone loss and fractures and can lead to osteoporosis. Therefore, it's particularly important for women to watch their protein intake.

Many athletes now stay away from high-protein diets—they cannot use protein for fuel; only carbohydrates and fats. And since high-protein diets will overtax the kidneys, which must dissolve the substances the body can't use in water and excrete them, excess protein can lead to dehydration.

Finally, excess protein is stored as fat. Overweight people run higher risks of developing certain types of cancer, high blood pressure, diabetes, and heart disease.

How much, then, is too much? A general rule of thumb for anyone age 19 or over is to multiply the ideal body weight by 0.36 to determine the daily requirement in grams. Therefore, a 120-pound woman will require 43 grams of protein daily. That goal can be reached in no time. For example, 1 cup of high-protein spaghetti has 13 grams, 1/2 cup of cottage cheese has 15 grams, and 3 ounces of canned tuna has 24.4 grams. Ultimately, protein consumption should be about 20 percent of your daily intake.

Fats: Easy to Store, Hard to Lose

"Fat" is the dietary word that sends shivers up our spines. With good reason; as with protein, we eat way too much fat. Most of the fat we eat has no nutritional value. And it's hard for the body to use it up.

Yet, there are some good fats. And some fat in our diet is important for good health. Fat helps support vital organs and provides insulation under our skin against extreme temperatures. Fat prevents dryness in the skin and hair. Most hormones are made from fats, and fats are required for vitamin and mineral absorption.

But we don't need much fat to survive. One tablespoon of vegetable oil a day would satisfy our dietary needs. Unfortunately, most of us consume much more than that. And too much fat can led to obesity and heart disease and contribute to certain types of cancers, particularly breast and colon cancer.

The major culprit involved in these diseases is cholesterol, which is a form of fat found in the blood. Cholesterol is used to manufacture hormones, but even if you eat no cholesterol, the body can make all it needs. Excess unused cholesterol can form fatty deposits on blood vessels and arteries, leading to a heart attack or stroke.

Saturated fats (those that are hard at room temperature, like butter, lard or coconut oil) will increase the amount of cholesterol in your blood. On the other hand, unsaturated fats, which are oils at room temperature, can help lower your cholesterol level and, for many people, help reduce the risk of developing heart disease. These fats come in two types, the mono-unsaturated, such as olive and peanut oils, and the polyunsaturated, such as safflower, corn, and cottonseed oils. Recently, fish oils have been found to protect against heart disease. These are commonly known as omega-3 fatty acids or EPA and are abundant in tuna, salmon, swordfish, bluefish, mackerel, and herring, as well as other fatty fish.

Regardless of the type of oil, too much fat is still dangerous. It's best to try to cut as much fat as possible out of our diets, keeping total intake to 20 to 30 percent of daily calories, and to limit cholesterol intake to 300 milligrams.

A daily menu with about 300 milligrams of cholesterol might include 1 cup of low-fat milk, ½ cup of cottage cheese, 1 tablespoon of butter, 3 ounces of chicken white meat, 3 ounces of veal, and 1 cup of egg noodles—and unlimited quantities of grains, vegetables, and fruits, which have no cholesterol.

Certain foods are so fatty that they'll blow your fat budget. Egg yolks, for example, have recently become a dietary no-no. Each egg yolk has 252 milligrams of cholesterol, and the American Heart Association suggests we eat no more than four eggs a week. It's also important to avoid such fatty foods as sour and heavy cream, mayonnaise, avocado, nuts, skin of chicken, hard cheeses, premium ice creams, cakes made with butter and egg yolks, gravy, and most luncheon meats.

Carbohydrates: High-Octane Energy

Not too long ago, people who wanted to lose weight were advised to keep away from starches such as bread, pasta, and potatoes. But as science has learned more about the way the body burns different types of foods, this recommendation has changed. That's good news for me, because I've always considered spaghetti with tomato sauce and a sprinkling of Parmesan cheese the ideal family meal: it's quick and easy to make, and even picky eaters love it.

We now know that complex carbohydrates, or starches (as opposed to simple carbohydrates, or sugars), actually are the best foods we can eat. They are clean, high-octane fuel that our bodies burn most efficiently for energy. And up to a third of the calories from complex carbohydrates come from its fiber, which we don't absorb.

Complex carbohydrates, such as potatoes, pasta, rice, bulgur, corn, dried beans and peas, and fruits and vegetables, are simply your best food friends. Their reputation for being fattening comes from what we put on them (butter, sour cream, and rich creamy sauces, for example). The truth is that our bodies use up more of the calories from complex carbohydrates than from proteins, and therefore they provide the best form of energy. Carbohydrates also are a healthier source of protein, with less fat and more vitamins and minerals. A diet high in carbohydrates can protect against heart disease and certain types of cancer, and can lower blood cholesterol levels and help stabilize blood sugar levels.

The other reason to load up on carbohydrates is that they actually help you lose weight and keep it off. Carbohydrates are metabolized into glucose, which is the substance our bodies use for energy. Low-carbohydrate diets actually are bad for us, because they don't provide enough glucose to feed the brain and muscles. Glucose is not stored in the brain; therefore, a glucose deficiency will result in fatigue, irritability, even depression. And when our blood sugar level drops, we naturally rush out in search of a quick fix— a candy bar, for instance—that will quickly restore our energy. Eating a balanced high-carbohydrate diet maintains your energy level and keeps you away from wild binges.

Fiber, the indigestible part of carbohydrates, is the dietary gold mine that does more than just fill you up. Fibrous foods take longer to digest and fill you up more quickly than other foods. The fiber then passes through the intestine, and helps clean out the bowel.

High-fiber, high-carbohydrate diets can not only make you healthy, they can keep you that way. Fiber has been shown to reduce obesity, high blood pressure, and high cholesterol levels— all important risk factors in heart disease. And starchy foods appear to protect us against certain types of cancer, especially colon and breast cancer, by binding to cancer-causing chemicals in the intestine and eliminating them. The National Cancer Institute has begun to study the effects of certain complex carbohydrates, particularly fresh fruits and vegetables, on risks of cancer.

With so much good news about carbohydrates, it's strange that the typical American diet still falls short on this wonder food. We should be getting 50 to 70 percent of our daily calories from carbohydrates.

So load up on pasta, vegetables, fruits, grains, beans, and salads as the bulk of your meal and you'll be surprised at how quickly your appetite is satisfied, how few hunger pangs you feel throughout the day, how much energy you have, and how quickly you start to shed unwanted pounds. And keep them off.

Sugar, Spice, and Everything Nice

Along with overdoses of fat and protein, there are two major diet-busters: salt and sugar. Salt and sugar lurk everywhere. They're hidden in just about all processed foods, and most of us have learned to love their taste and, unwittingly, have become addicted to them. Both are acquired tastes and have virtually no nutritional value. And they can actually do us harm—particularly salt.

Despite the hoopla over its danger, salt, which can lead to high blood pressure, heart disease, and stroke, is still the leading food additive. Because there is enough salt in the natural foods we eat, not to mention the overload in processed foods, we'd need to add only about 1/10 teaspoon daily to satisfy our body's natural need. But in our society, it's not hard to get more than 3 to 4 teaspoons a day.

People who have high blood pressure or are hereditarily predisposed to it should dramatically reduce their salt intake. But no one needs excess salt. It only increases fluid retention, which impedes weight loss. And for women, it can aggravate symptoms of premenstrual syndrome.

Because salt is an acquired taste, it's best to eliminate it slowly. Once you've gotten used to less salt, you'll probably find your food tastes better without it.

Unlike salt, sugar is a food—it is a simple carbohydrate. But like salt, sugar feeds our taste buds and psychological needs rather than our physiological needs. Sugar has become the instinctive reward, the dietary no-no that we secretly, or not so secretly, crave. But sugar is nothing but empty calories, and most sweet foods are laden with fat.

Sugar plays havoc with your energy level (and hence your moods) and is particularly dangerous for dieters. Because sugar requires little processing, it is quickly absorbed into our bloodstreams, giving us that quick pick-me-up. However, as our blood sugar level rises, the pancreas releases the hormone insulin to lower it. The more blood sugar we have, the more insulin is released and the faster our blood sugar level drops. When it drops too low, which it can easily do a few hours after a sugar binge, we feel tired, irritable, and hungry, and crave more sugar—which only exacerbates the cycle.

If sugar's not good for me, you say, how about artificial sweeteners? Artificial sweeteners do you no good in the long run. They only perpetuate your love affair with sweets; in fact, they even increase your appetite for them. How many times have you seen obese people in the supermarket with shopping carts filled with dietary foods?

Sugar, like salt, is an acquired taste. If you start to reduce it from your diet gradually, you'll probably find you don't miss it after a while. And once you get away from sugar, you'll soon find that sweet processed foods simply are too sweet.

The good news is that there are things you can add to foods to greatly enhance their flavors without threatening your health or your waistline. For example, 2 teaspoons of cinnamon sprinkled on an apple before baking packs a flavor wallop. So does a cup of fresh basil chopped into tomato sauce. Assertive seasoning is one sure way to make eating a pleasure while you're losing weight. Weaning your taste buds away from sugar and salt and toward more flavor is also a big help in portion control. Often, sugar and salt addicts keep eating simply to get more of these tastes. You're much less likely to crave more cinnamon, or basil, and, therefore, more likely to simply stop eating when you're no longer hungry.

Caffeine is another addictive substance that can interfere with healthy living. If you have a problem with nervousness, tension, or falling asleep, a switch to decaffeinated coffee, tea, and soft drinks may act like magic in resolving these symptoms. True caffeine addicts may find themselves with powerful headaches if they try to eliminate the substance completely. One woman I know compromises by allowing herself two cups of regular coffee in the morning, and no more caffeine for the rest of the day.

Gaining control over the amount of sugar, salt, and caffeine in your diet is an excellent way to begin a weight-loss plan. Whether the cutbacks are drastic or moderate, the increased sense of personal control will help empower you to make other healthy choices.

The Meals

We do not sit down at the table and eat carbohydrates, fats, and proteins. Rather, we eat foods that combine many different types of nutrients. And getting the mix right, in combinations that please you and slim you, is what successful dieting is all about.

Let me say from the outset that I don't believe in absolute or complicated diet plans; I don't think you have to weigh your food or divide it into strictly defined metric servings, and I certainly take exception to the unscientific diets that hold that rotating kiwis and oranges does something magical to your waistline. Just because a diet program is complicated does not make it more precise or more scientific. Following some of the programs I've seen described in magazines and diet books requires a degree in engineering! To my mind, the harder a program is to remember and follow, the less likely it is to work.

Still, I *do* believe that each person needs guidelines, especially those who have never dieted before. In the next chapter, I include several exercises aimed at helping you develop diet strategies. But here, to help you start out and lose that initial (and encouraging) few pounds, I'm going to give you some sample outlines and menus.

The Happy Eater Plan

This low-calorie, high-energy eating plan is designed for an average-size woman who wants to lose weight. Men may need to double the servings of grains and vegetables in order to feel comfortably full, but protein servings should not be increased.

I've broken this down into the classic three-meal-a-day eating pattern. But you can, if you choose, spread the servings into more frequent meals, or save a fruit or grain from one meal to use as a between-meal snack.

Serving Sizes:

Grain serving: 1 slice bread; 1 muffin; ½ cup pasta; ½ cup rice

Protein serving: 3 ounces lean chicken, turkey, veal, pork, or beef; 1 egg; 1 cup skim milk; ½ cup yogurt or cottage cheese

Fruit serving: 1 apple, pear, or peach; 1 cup cherries or strawberries; ½ grapefruit; ½ banana; 1 tablespoon raisins

Vegetables: 1 potato a day; ½ cup peas, beans, corn a day; unlimited quantities of other vegetables at any meal, or between meals

Meal Plan

Breakfast

1 fruit
1 grain (cereal or bread)
1 low-fat dairy product (low-fat milk or yogurt)
(add 1 egg, twice a week, if desired)

Lunch

2 grains
1 meat or low-fat dairy product
2 or more vegetables
1 fruit

Dinner

2 grains
1 protein
1 low-fat dairy product (optional)
2 or more vegetables
1 fruit

Breakfast

When I was on fad diets, I ate nothing but a piece of fruit and a cup of coffee for breakfast. I wasn't that hungry when I awoke, and it seemed like a good opportunity to save calories. The problem was, I never felt fully awake; I used to tell people I wasn't a "morning person." And by midmorning I was hungry, irritable, and too busy with patients to stop and snack. So I began to add a bran muffin to my breakfast. And lo and behold, I found that I could sail through the morning feeling energetic and alert and feel not a growl in my stomach until noon. As it turns out, I *am* a morning person.

Breakfast is the fuel we need to get us going in the morning; if you skip this meal, you'll feel it for the rest of the day. Your low blood sugar could set off food cravings that could, in turn, trigger binges.

Still, if you're a person who's never hungry in the morning, don't try to cram down a lot of food anyway. Instead, try eating a small breakfast at, say, 10:30 a.m., after you've been at work for a while.

Breakfast does not have to be a big or heavy meal. Except for Sunday brunch, I prefer a whole-grain muffin or cereal to pancakes. But, most important, getting off to a good start means getting plenty of carbohydrates.

Here are some suggestions to start you off:

Breakfast #1

½ grapefruit
1 serving cereal (such as Grape Nuts, Muesli, oatmeal) with low-fat milk
Decaffeinated coffee or tea

Breakfast #2

1 cup low-fat yogurt mixed with a banana, kiwi, or other fresh fruit, and 1 tablespoon wheat germ
1 piece whole-wheat toast with a little sugar-free jam or apple butter
Decaffeinated coffee or tea

Breakfast #3

½ cantaloupe or other seasonal fresh fruit
1 whole wheat or pumpernickel English muffin with natural peanut butter
Café au lait (made with decaffeinated coffee and hot low-fat milk)

Breakfast #4

6 ounces fruit juice
1 poached egg
1 piece whole wheat toast
Café au lait or plain decaffeinated coffee or tea

Breakfast #5

Fruit or fruit juice
2 pieces French toast (made with 1 egg, low-fat milk, cinnamon, and nutmeg)
Decaffeinated coffee or tea

Lunch

Do you hit a slump in the mid-to-late afternoon? Do you come home from work totally beat? Although it's natural to have less energy late in the day, I find I can even out the peaks and valleys if I make sure I eat a very nutritious lunch.

Lunch doesn't have to be your biggest meal of the day (though this may be ideal for weight loss and it's something I often experiment with on vacations and weekends, when my schedule permits). But the lunches here are designed for workday meals, eaten on the run, and often at restaurants. They all include plenty of carbohydrates.

Lunch #1

2 vegetable burritos (made with corn tortillas, beans, vegetables, and low-fat cheese)
Fresh fruit or frozen yogurt

Lunch #2

Pasta salad (made with spinach or tomato pasta, chick-peas or tuna, lots of vegetables, basil, and reduced-oil or oil-free salad dressing)
Raisin pumpernickel roll
Fruit juice spritzer

Lunch #3

Curried carrot soup
Tabouli salad
½ pita with hummus
Fresh fruit

Lunch #4

Vegetarian pizza
Tossed salad with reduced-oil or oil-free salad dressing
Fresh fruit

Lunch #5

Chicken salad (made with chicken breast, broccoli, red pepper,
   scallion, dill, and light mayonnaise mixed with low-fat yogurt)
Apple or bran muffin
Fresh orange juice spritzer

Dinner

In our house, as in most American homes, dinner is the meal we
look forward to, that we savor and linger over. The whole family
is often together at this time, and on days when we have sufficient
luck and patience we use the meal to reestablish our closeness
rather than to scold the children.

Now that I prepare healthy, lighter foods, I make a special effort
to make the meal look colorful and attractive by using foods of
contrasting colors, lots of fresh herbs, and sliced fruit as garnishes.
And I've found that if I eat meals higher in carbohydrates than in
proteins and fats, I wake the next morning feeling much more
refreshed.

A fruit dessert is included in the meal plans here. But I should
confess that in our house, it's usually not eaten with the dinner. By
the time we get to dessert the children are usually anxious to leave
the table. So I let them eat their dessert whenever they wish in the
evening. And my husband and I enjoy ours in bed as a pre-sleep
treat.

Dinner #1

Cream of broccoli soup (made with broccoli, leeks, celery, gar-
   lic, chicken broth, and low-fat milk)
Broiled tuna steak, sprinkled with lemon juice and fresh herbs
Roast new potatoes
Carrots and zucchini, steamed with parsley or mint
Fresh berries with low-fat lemon yogurt

Dinner #2

Chicken couscous
Frozen low-fat yogurt

Dinner #3

Vegetarian lasagna
Tossed green salad, with reduced-oil or oil-free salad dressing
Sourdough roll
Poached pears

Dinner #4

Cold sesame noodles
Stir-fry vegetables with chicken, shrimp, or scallops
Brown rice
Orange slices

Dinner #5

Endive and asparagus salad
Broiled chicken fillet, marinaded in rosemary, garlic, and a little
  olive oil
Fettuccine tossed with steamed julienne carrots and zucchini
  with lots of fresh parsley, basil, or dill
Apple tart (made with one whole wheat pie crust)

Happy eating!

11

Eating and You

During the first year that I quit fad diets and began walking, I spent a good deal of time researching the "right" foods to eat. If you've read the previous chapter, you, too, now know that concentrating on carbohydrates—pasta, brown rice, bread, and, especially, large quantities of all kinds of fruits and vegetables—is the secret of healthy eating. Add some low-fat dairy products and small servings of meat, chicken, and fish, and you've got the perfect eating plan.

But knowing what to eat is a far cry from actually eating it. So the next hurdle I faced, after my nutrition research, was integrating what I learned into my daily food shopping, cooking, home eating, and restaurant eating habits. What I discovered, to my surprise, was that the habit-building techniques I had developed to make walking a part of my life were rather easily applied to healthy eating.

The exercises in this chapter will help you build on the skills you've already accumulated by becoming a regular, happy walker. For healthy eating to work in the long run, and result in weight loss that is sustained for a lifetime, it has to become a natural, easy part of your everyday life.

Becoming a healthy eater does not mean that you won't *ever* eat chocolate cake again. If you're like me, a diet that strict would make you feel deprived, persecuted, and rebellious. When I succeeded in getting my weight down to 120 pounds and keeping it there for six months, I decided I would indulge in a few bites of outrageous sweets once or twice a year, when faced with some truly delicious dessert. But I was careful not to let these exceptions become the rule again. Whenever I deviate from healthy eating, I climb right back onto the plan the very next meal.

Healthy eating should become your rule—the meal pattern you fall back on, time and again, after minor deviations. The goal is to make it as much a habit as taking a walk four or five times a week. Choosing healthy foods that you genuinely like to eat is the key to forming this habit. Some of these foods you no doubt already like. Some will be newly acquired tastes.

To apply the diet basics and eating plan in the last chapter to your own life-style requires that you take at least a quick glance at how and what you're eating now. You may be relieved to know that I'm not going to ask you to keep an "eating diary." I know that's a favorite technique of dietitians, and I'm sure people who keep such diaries learn a lot from them. But if you're like me when I was overeating, you don't want to directly confront what you're actually putting in your mouth.

The exercise that follows is a somewhat gentler way of increasing your eating awareness. It helps you define your personal eating obstacles. After the exercise I suggest some specific strategies for preparing for the problems that are bound to lie ahead.

Exercise 1

Check off the obstacles you're likely to face when you try to change your eating habits.

1. _____ I feel hungry.
2. _____ I forget I'm on a diet.
3. _____ I give in to temptation when eating with others.
4. _____ I lose my willpower after the first drink of wine.

5. _____ I eat too much in restaurants.
6. _____ I want to avoid wasting food.
7. _____ I cook for my family, who resist diet meals.
8. _____ I cheat when I'm tired.
9. _____ I feel depressed when I weigh myself and see no progress.
10. _____ I eat very quickly.
11. _____ I forget to drink enough fluids.
12. _____ I eat while watching television.
13. _____ I eat standing up over the sink.
14. _____ I am teased by family members or friends.
15. _____ I overeat during periods of stress.
16. _____ I feel embarrassed if people know I'm dieting.

If I had taken the exercise above before I started my Happy Eater plan, I probably would have checked every one of the listed obstacles to healthy eating. These obstacles are, indeed, formidable. But as with the obstacles to acquiring a walking habit that we analyzed in Chapter 5, you can arm yourself against them by thinking through, in advance, how you'll handle the situation. Let's take a look at them, one by one.

1. I feel hungry.

When a person without a weight problem says "I'm hungry," or even "I'm starving," he or she is generally experiencing an uncomfortably hollow sensation in the stomach, or, in extreme cases, a sharp, intermittent pain and a feeling of light-headedness.

When an overweight person on a diet says "I'm hungry," however, it may have little to do with sensations in the stomach. What the dieter really means is "I feel deprived" or "I would like to eat more, or different, foods than I'm 'supposed to.' "

On the Happy Eater plan you should *never* feel hungry after a meal, though, to be honest, you may well feel deprived on occasion. If you do feel actual hunger, you simply need to eat more. The meal plan allows for unlimited quantities of most cooked and raw vegetables. If you serve these in abundance at every meal, sprinkled with lemon or large quantities of dried or fresh herbs, you'll always be able to eat until you're full.

If what you're feeling is deprived, however, another plateful of steamed carrots with basil may *not* be what you need. Look back at the discussion of rewards in Chapter 6. When you're feeling deprived, take a "me break" and do something nice for yourself. Light some candles, turn on a favorite record, and waltz around the living room repeating your affirmations: "I have good qualities; I have important, caring relationships; I have scored some emotional victories; I'm gaining some control over my need for food; I am a success."

Chances are your "hunger" will disappear before your 15-minute "me break" is over.

2. I forget I'm on a diet.

I've been obsessed with my weight for so long that I seldom actually forget that I'm supposed to be eating healthy. But Rosann, the 26-year-old receptionist in my podiatry office, says one of her problems is that she doesn't remember what she's supposed to eat until *after* she's downed an order of french-fried onion rings or a handful of cookies.

That's why there are currently yellow Post-It notes that say "Lose 10 Pounds," "Take a Walk," and "Eat Those Carbos" near the photocopy machine and the telephones and in the ladies' room. Rosann has found this is a great method of remembering her vows and reinforcing her determination. And, yes, she is looking quite a bit slimmer lately.

3. I give in to temptation when eating with others.

When everyone around me is ordering martinis, prime rib, and chocolate mud pie, it's not easy to tell the waiter to bring me a wine spritzer, grilled tuna, and fresh strawberries, hold the whipped cream. And it's even harder to maintain a cheery attitude while watching my friends casually indulging in all the foods I used to eat.

Like most people, I hate feeling left out—isolated from a group of happy, animated people I long to be part of. It brings back old childhood and adolescent bruises: the day I got chosen last for volleyball; the party I wasn't invited to; the "in crowd" in high school that wouldn't accept me.

Until your new healthy eating habit becomes strong, it's a good idea to keep away from situations in which others will be overindulging. If you do need to attend such occasions—and I'm certainly not suggesting you miss a wedding celebration or cancel business lunches—try to decide in advance what you'll order.

The bright side of this picture is that today more people than ever before are trying to eat healthfully. In many business circles, bottled water, not martinis, is the standard order. So be brave and order what you know you should. You're more likely to excite admiration than pity in those around you.

4. I lose my willpower after the first drink of wine.

Many people find that complete abstinence from alcohol leads to the quickest possible weight loss. Not only do you save the 100 calories or so in each glass of wine, but you aren't tempted by that soft, easygoing, alcoholic haze to start nibbling at the bowl of mixed nuts at the bar.

If you do decide to drink, choose carefully and sip slowly. Try waiting to drink until after you've ordered and your food arrives. When the waiter asks for your drink order, get some club soda and lime for a starter, and then order wine to arrive with your meal. Always ask for a glass of water, too. Wine, gin or vodka with juice, or "straight up" drinks have many fewer calories than heavily sweetened drinks such as margaritas or frozen daiquiris.

5. I eat too much in restaurants.

I've noticed a new eating pattern among my friends. We're very careful about what we cook and eat at home, but lose all perspective as soon as we're in a restaurant. If you only eat out once every month or two, this is probably not going to ruin your health or your weight-loss program. But if you eat out frequently, learning to order correctly in restaurants is a necessity.

The problem is that foods that seem healthy—such as broiled fish, salads, or fruit-based desserts—may arrive swimming in fat, sugar, or salt. Large serving sizes and unwanted courses can lure us into eating more than we should. And it's hard to find nutritionally sound meals in places that give quick service like delis and fast-food restaurants.

Here are some ways to handle this problem. For breakfasts out, choose cooked or cold cereal or a whole-grain muffin—*not* eggs, bacon, or sausage. Then, so you don't feel deprived, also order something you usually don't have at home: perhaps fresh orange juice, a fruit salad, or half a cantaloupe.

For quick lunches, try salad bars in fast-food restaurants, and go easy on the dressing. Avoid the selections that are premixed with mayonnaise or salad dressing. A plain hamburger or a meatless pizza makes a satisfying lunch. In delis, try a turkey sandwich on whole-wheat bread, hold the mayo, or a vegetable salad and a toasted whole-grain bagel. Take advantage of the great salad bars in oriental markets.

Try not to go out for dinner when you're famished. Have a small snack first to enhance your self-control. When I eat dinner out I almost always order broiled or poached fish. I've never learned to cook fish really well at home, and so I find eating it out a treat. These days the waiters aren't surprised if I ask for no butter on the fish or vegetables, or sauces and salad dressings on the side.

In virtually every restaurant you can order a salad as an appetizer, which is a great way to start the meal. While you're waiting you can eat one unbuttered roll or piece of bread to help fill you up. I always order à la carte rather than choosing the full dinner. The dinner price may seem like a bargain but if you eat more than you want to, it's a poor bargain. I also avoid buffets unless my willpower is particularly strong; the array of food is just too tempting.

If you eat out frequently, keep your eyes open for restaurants with low-calorie or "heart healthy" items on the menus. In our neighborhood there's a Chinese restaurant that serves a variety of vegetable, shrimp, and chicken dishes steamed with wine. Italian restaurants can be relied on to have a selection of healthy pasta with marinara sauce, and many also serve steamed mussels, clams, or mixed seafood soups and pasta dishes that you can enjoy. If I want dessert, I choose a fresh fruit or sorbet, an ice made with water rather than cream. But most often I skip dessert in the restaurant and have my poached fruit at home in bed.

6. I want to avoid wasting food.

"Don't feel bad if you buy lots of fruits and vegetables and then you end up going out to dinner a lot that week and the produce gets spoiled. What have you wasted—six or eight dollars? Think of what one day in the cardiac care unit costs!" When Annette Waupeha, a registered dietitian in private practice in New York, shared this bit of advice with me, I decided to stop worrying about throwing out limp carrots, rotten lettuce, and overripe tomatoes.

It's far better to keep an overabundance of fresh things in the house, so you'll always have something healthy to prepare, than to worry about waste and face an empty refrigerator in the evening. And, please, let's give up the "clean plate ethic" and stop worrying about finishing up every bit of food on our plates.

How can a responsible person throw away perfectly good food? Well, here's news: easily. If your hunger is satisfied and there's still food on your plate, just let it sit there. If you want to do something to alleviate world hunger, send a contribution to a worthy cause.

7. I cook for my family, who resist diet meals.

Your children and spouse do not have to eat the same foods you do. Nor do you have to abandon your eating plan. If you're the cook and you have the time and energy to prepare two different meals, fine. Usually you won't, of course. But if you look closely at the food plan you'll probably see many things on it that even your set of picky eaters will like. Minor modifications can make the plan suit both healthy and not-yet-ready-for-health eaters. For example, you can serve butter on their vegetables or pasta, and not on your own. You can heap your plate with salad, steamed vegetables, and a small piece of chicken, while they eat mostly chicken and avoid the vegetables.

When the rest of the family wants to eat a food that is simply not on your diet and there's no alternative, don't get hung up in guilt. Simply eat the least-fattening foods available or eat smaller portions than usual. Then go back to your own food plan at the next meal.

8. I cheat when I'm tired.

This is a common problem among people who work too hard. It's the end of a long, difficult day. There are dozens of important things still undone. And you're too tired to move. In fact, the only thing you have energy for is standing in front of the refrigerator and cramming things into your mouth.

I know from bitter experience that binge eating in moments of great exhaustion is not a satisfying experience. I barely taste the food, and certainly don't enjoy it, physically or emotionally. It's more a form of punishment than pleasure.

If you expect evening exhaustion to be a problem, prepare something healthy that you *can* guiltlessly stuff yourself with when you get home. When I'm in this state, I like to eat raw vegetables perhaps picked up on the way home, already cleaned, from a salad bar with a low-cal dip. (My favorite is a simple combination of low-fat yogurt, 2 tablespoons of curry, and a good dash of cumin and Tabasco sauce. It socks a big flavor, and the vegetables give me something to chew while I calm down and decide what I really want to eat.) Drinking a glass of water can also help calm the appetite.

9. I feel depressed when I weigh myself and see no progress.

Here's a radical notion: get rid of your bathroom scale. You don't have to throw it out, but you can place it in the back of a closet somewhere, out of sight. The best way to lose weight and keep it off over the long term is to reduce intake of fats and proteins in a moderate, gradual, and permanent way. It's a long road, and you can drive yourself crazy if you keep looking for road signs every day.

The self-esteem of too many women I know rides on the number that comes up when they step on that scale each morning. As you and I know, daily weigh-ins can be pretty disappointing. What's more important and more useful is how you *feel* when you lose weight and gradually get into shape through walking.

So forget the scale, and get used to looking at yourself in a full-length mirror every day. The more often you look at yourself, and the more honest (and not overly critical) you are in your appraisal, the better able you'll be to deal honestly with yourself. Soon you'll be able to recognize your good features as well as your bad ones. You'll see changes in your weight and well-being. Trust me: as it happens, you won't need a scale. You'll *know* it.

10. I eat very quickly.

This is a tough habit to break. I have one friend who's trained himself to put down his fork between bites, chew thoroughly, and take a few breaths before he picks his fork back up. That's a great method of letting your stomach register what you've already eaten before you plunge in for more.

Another way to slow down is to pace yourself with a friend or relative who eats slowly. Copy this person through a meal or two, pausing when he or she does. You might find the new rhythm quite pleasant. When you eat quickly, you tend to swallow great gulps of air along with your food, which can lead to a gassy, uncomfortable stomach later on. But the major benefit of eating slowly is that the meal lasts longer! We've established that eating is among the most pleasurable experiences in life. Why rush through it?

11. I forget to drink enough fluids.

If you're very busy during the day, it's easy to neglect drinking. Drinking eight or more glasses of water a day flushes fats from the body and helps you lose weight quicker. It also keeps your skin, hair, and nails in good condition and prevents the light-headed feeling that comes from dehydration.

Try keeping a thermos of water on your desk as you work. Herbal teas and fruit juice mixed with club soda are other good choices. Many companies make calorie-free flavored waters that are welcome treats for healthy eaters.

12. I eat while watching television.

It's best to avoid eating while doing something that has your mind distracted—like reading, working, or watching TV. I know this is a hard one to change, but think about how *unconscious* eating becomes when you're involved in something else. Have you ever spent an evening watching a video and then looked down at an empty bowl with little memory of how and when that popcorn disappeared? Why miss out on the pleasure?

As a general rule, I try to avoid between-meal eating. I don't even like to visit the kitchen except when I'm preparing a meal. Walking through seems to put the idea of eating into my mind. But if I'm really yearning to nibble sometimes, I don't fight it. I prepare myself a large plate of raw vegetables and chew away!

13. I eat standing up over the sink.

Am I the only one who does this? I know the best idea is to set a lovely table and enjoy the ritual of a pleasant meal, even if I'm eating by myself. But there are times when I'm overwhelmed by the desire to stand at the kitchen sink and gulp down some food. So, I do it. I just make sure the food is something good for me and tasty. For example, cottage cheese, a little chopped onion, and a slice of tomato on a low-salt cracker, topped with black pepper, makes a good, crunchy, mouth-satisfying lunch. And the crumbs go right in the sink and are easy to clean up!

14. I am teased by family members or friends.

"Oh no, do you eat healthy *too?* How perfect do you want to be?"

"Grilled fish, eh? Why don't you order something with more cholesterol?"

"You're thin enough. It's time to relax."

Those are just some of the nonsupportive remarks I hear when I'm eating with others who, in fact, are envious of my habit of making healthy food choices. Reread the discussion in Chapter 5 of finding people to support your walking habit. You'll need to use the same methods to find people who support healthy eating.

15. I overeat during periods of stress.

By my personal definition, stress is worrying, the mental rerunning of the "I should have said" and "I forgot to do" of the work or family problems during my relaxation time. Overeating when this type of tape is running in my mind does not bring the slow, delicious pleasure of, say, deciding to indulge in cake because today's my birthday. Like eating when I'm overexhausted, it's more a form of punishment than pleasure.

Here's a time when going for a walk serves a double purpose. It gives you time to focus on the source of your stress and run that tape until you're bored and finished with it. And it gets you far away from food until you've calmed down.

When you're feeling stressed, put on those walking shoes. If you've already taken a walk that day, take another one. You deserve to feel better!

16. I feel embarrassed if people know I'm dieting.

I *never* tell people I'm dieting. "These are the foods I like to eat," I tell any inquirers. Most of the time, it turns out, they're not interested in making fun of me but in acquiring some good habits for themselves. But I don't feel I have to be an apostle of good eating for everyone. For although healthy eating is excellent for your mind and body, it's not necessarily the most scintillating topic of conversation. I don't want to become a food bore.

So when someone says: "Oh, you've lost weight! How did you do it?" I sometimes just acknowledge the compliment with a smile and switch the conversation to the latest movie or newspaper headline.

LEARNING TO LOVE THE FOODS THAT LOVE YOU

Most overweight people, I've found, have certain foods that trigger overeating. It's best to identify these enemies clearly and adopt a battle plan for dealing with them. They'll probably never be vanquished. But you can reach a kind of détente in which you avoid confronting the enemy, but never give it a chance to again take over your life.

The following exercise will help you identify your personal food enemies.

Exercise 2

Check off the items that you expect to have the most trouble limiting or eliminating.

1. _____ sugar
2. _____ ice cream, cakes, candies
3. _____ artificial sweeteners (diet soda, etc.)
4. _____ salt use
5. _____ salty snacks (potato chips, etc.)

6. _____ butter
7. _____ cooking oils and fats
8. _____ salad dressings and gravies
9. _____ eggs
10. _____ size of meat portions
11. _____ number of meat servings a day
12. _____ cream or half-and-half in coffee
13. _____ regular milk
14. _____ cheese
15. _____ fried foods
16. _____ quantities of all foods
17. _____ quantities of certain foods (be specific) _____
_____
18. _____ other (be specific) _____

In weaning yourself from unhealthy, fattening foods, it's a good idea to tackle one major problem at a time. For most people, the biggest food temptation falls into either the sugary or salty snack group. If one of these is your nemesis, work on it first, and then gradually move on to correcting other food habits. Let's look at the items in logical groups:

1, 2, 3: Conquering the Sweet Tooth

Joan had just turned 39, that crucial birthday when everyone realizes that 40 is just around the corner. A partner in a wholesale video equipment business with her husband, Joan has had a weight problem all her life. Her height is 5 feet 5; she formerly weighed 180 pounds and wore a "size 14 going on 16" dress. Now, at 42, she's a size 8 and weighs 137. She's been on a healthy eating plan for two years, but she didn't adopt the whole program in one step.

"My big eating problem could be summed up in one word: cake," Joan told me. If there was cake in the house (and she made sure there was), she ate it—all of it—usually secretly, around midnight, after her husband went to bed.

The first thing Joan did to conquer her weight problem was to begin walking. She had to start at the beginner's level, since she was so out of shape. "After a couple of months, the walking gave me confidence to do what I knew I needed to do—completely stop eating cake." She ate other foods as she liked, but she banned sweets from the house and enlisted her husband's help to keep her from indulging when friends ordered cake in restaurants. "He held my hand under the table, winked at me, whispered romantic comments. He was great at distracting me," she says.

It took three months for Joan's craving for sweets to subside completely, but during that time she learned to eat lots of canned pineapple and poached fruit, which she found satisfied her sweet tooth. As the craving diminished, she found even the poached fruit tasted rather sweet, and now mixes it with low-fat yogurt.

"After I conquered the cake thing, I knew I could really lose weight. I was up to the intermediate walking level and felt a lot stronger. I had lost only about 8 pounds from eliminating sweets, but the rest came off more quickly as I ate healthier foods."

Sugar addictions, like Joan's, are incredibly common. Not only do cakes, candy, and ice cream add weight in themselves, but they send your mood and energy levels soaring and dipping unpredictably in the hours after you eat them. So a few hours after you've eaten something sugary, your blood sugar falls rapidly, and with it, your mood and energy level. Many people respond to that dip by craving yet more sugar. This dangerous cycle leads to obesity and a feeling of being out of control.

If you're addicted to sugar, I think it's very important to keep satisfying your sweet tooth—but in ways that are healthier for your body. Sugar addicts should *not* eliminate desserts from their lives. Instead, they should have small servings of frozen yogurt, ice milk, or sorbet at the time of day they used to eat cake and premium ice cream. Raw or poached fruit cooked in water and frozen apple or orange juice concentrate (not sugar and water) are other sweet dessert alternatives.

Artificially sweetened food—like low-calorie cocoa and diet soda—are okay on occasion, but if used frequently they only perpetuate your longing for sweets. Soft drinks contain large amounts of phosphorus, which causes the body to excrete calcium. *And* they perpetuate cravings for sugar.

Here are some more tips for breaking the sugar habit:

- Buy unsweetened cereals and add fresh fruit or raisins.
- For special occasions, bake your own cookies, cakes, and pies. Reduce the sugar in the recipes by half, adding instead raisins or nuts, or sweeten with a little fruit juice.
- Buy plain low-fat yogurt and mix in fresh fruit or unsweetened fruit butters.
- Instead of sodas, drink club soda mixed with a little fruit juice or a slice of lemon or lime.
- Get children off to the right start early. Don't give them sweets as treats.

4, 5: Bypassing the Salt Shaker

There are people who can wave away chocolate layer cake without regret, but can't resist a bowl of salty nuts or potato chips. These are usually the same folks who have a heavy hand with the salt shaker during meals.

Nature was particularly unfair to me. When I was overweight, I was addicted to both sugar and salt. I tackled the sugar problem first, but it wasn't until I reduced my salt intake that the pounds really began to drop off. Excess salt causes the body to retain water. This is particularly discouraging when you're trying to lose weight; even if you're doing everything else right, the excess salt can keep your waistband tight and the pounds on.

As with sugar, eliminating salt is best done gradually. One good method is to keep shakers full of other spices and herbs on the table when you eat so you can fulfill your urge to shake some flavor on your food. I particularly like to use shakers of premixed spices on my vegetables and salads. My favorites are Cajun and Italian seasoning mixes. I've also switched from condiments that are high in sodium, such as mustard, barbecue sauce, ketchup, and soy sauce, to the low-sodium products now available.

If you're used to using a lot of salt when you cook, try substituting other assertive seasonings. I like to double the amount of garlic and scallions in recipes to give a flavor wallop. I use four times the amount of dried tarragon, basil, parsley, and thyme recipes call for, and a full cup of fresh herbs when I have them. These can be used on popcorn, too, for some salt-free snacking. And do read the labels of the commercially prepared foods you buy; you'll find salt everywhere. When you have time, it's best to prepare things at home so you can control salt intake. Otherwise, opt for low-salt foods.

6, 7, 8: Out of the Fat Trap

While cutting back on sugar and salt is usually a major project, avoiding fats is something many people find easier to do. Drastically reducing the amount of butter and cooking oil you use is one of the quickest ways to lose weight.

The first step is to buy some inexpensive nonstick skillets and pans (and replace them when the finish begins to get worn out). Also buy a couple of pastry brushes. Then if you need to grease a pan, pour some oil into a small cup and brush it on. You'll use a lot less that way. I use very little butter, but when I do want the flavor, I brush some on the pan. Spray cans of corn oil are also useful.

Don't be afraid to experiment with leaving out large quantities of fat from recipes. The brand of turkey stuffing I use calls for 1/4 pound of melted butter. One day I simply left out the butter and added more chopped mushrooms, celery, garlic, and herbs. No one complained. Butter and oil can also be left out of rice and pasta recipes with little loss of taste.

To speed weight loss, sauté onions and garlic in a couple of tablespoons of water and wine instead of oil. If you let the liquid evaporate and keep stirring over a medium-high flame, you can actually brown the edges of the onions.

Salad dressings can add lots of fat and calories, but there are many commercial preparations that don't use any oil. Or make your own low-calorie versions, heavy on the vinegar and seasonings, light on the oil.

9, 10, 11, 12, 13, 14, 15: Cutting Cholesterol

If you're a bacon-and-eggs-for-breakfast person, a healthy eating plan will mean a major overhaul. So think carefully about what new healthy foods you'd like to try for breakfast. Canadian-style bacon has much less fat than the standard variety and makes a healthy substitute. And you may find that one egg is as satisfying as two. When making omelets or french toast, I use one whole egg and two egg whites. Yes, I throw the extra egg yolks down the drain. I still feel a little guilty for the "waste," but I'm getting used to it.

Some people who can switch to low-fat milk and yogurt without a problem in most situations desperately miss half-and-half or regular milk in their coffee. If this happens to you, carefully analyze your situation. If you drink only a cup or two of coffee in the morning, it may be worth the calories to use a dab of half-and-half or regular milk. I did this for the first year that I was dieting. Then I actually found it easier to give up the morning coffee and substitute a tall glass of half orange juice and half seltzer than to switch to skim milk in coffee. *Everyone* should be wary of those small, individual containers of "creamer" given out in delis and less expensive restaurants. They often contain high-cholesterol coconut oil. Ask the waitress for skim or regular milk instead.

Cheese lovers don't have to give it up, but they do need to choose lower-fat varieties. Farmers' cheese, goat cheese, low-fat cottage cheese, feta, and part-skim ricotta, mozzarella, Neufchatel, and Camembert are good choices. And experiment with the other low-fat cheeses now coming into the supermarkets.

If Southern fried chicken, french-fried potatoes, and fried won-tons are the types of foods you long for, soft, steamed, or boiled foods will not satisfy you. Instead, you need to search for methods and recipes that produce crunchy, crisp food *without* using a lot of oil. See the recipes later in this chapter for suggestions.

16, 17: Eating a Little Less

The sad truth is that as we get older our bodies tend to need less food. If at 30 we eat the exact same food we ate at 20, we'll probably gain weight. After 30, that same quantity will probably add about a pound a year. The gain is insidious. That's why many previously thin people wake up at 45 to find themselves 15 pounds overweight.

One way to eat less without suffering is to use more vegetables as filler in recipes. Three ounces of canned tuna expands gloriously when you add finely chopped carrot and celery. One scrambled egg may seem a paltry portion; but if you sauté a dozen mush-rooms, onions, and some basil with it, it will fill the plate nicely and be more satisfying. Half a chicken sandwich by itself can give you a "poor little dieter" feeling, but if you serve it up with a large salad and a cup of consommé you'll feel, instead, like an elegant diner.

After you've switched to a healthier diet and gotten used to the new eating pattern, you might consider speeding up your weight loss by reducing quantities. Eating slowly and consciously and leaving at least one or two bites on my plate when I've finished a meal are the methods I use to reduce quantity. Leaving food on my plate gives me a delicious sense of control. And getting up from the table as soon as I'm finished eating, rather than lingering over the leftovers, also helps me cut down on quantities.

MENU STRATEGIES

Now that you've considered your problem food areas, it's time to consider which healthy foods you already like. If you've never gone on a weight-loss diet before, it may take some experimenting before you can answer these questions. But with just a little thought, veteran dieters should be able to remember the foods they enjoyed on other diets.

EXERCISE 3

Which of the following healthy foods do you enjoy eating?

_____ raw salads
_____ fresh fruits (specify favorites): _____
_____ canned fruits (no sugar added; specify favorites): _____
_____

_____ brown rice
_____ bulgur
_____ tofu
_____ low-fat yogurt
_____ corn, safflower, canola, olive oil
_____ low-fat salad dressings
_____ steamed vegetables (specify favorites): _____
_____ low-fat cottage cheese
_____ "cream" soups made with low-fat milk
_____ broths and vegetable soups
_____ cereals (specify favorites): _____
_____ dips made with yogurt and/or cottage cheese
_____ spaghetti and other pastas
_____ bread, crackers, rolls
_____ tomato-based sauces
_____ broiled, steamed, or sautéed fish and shellfish (specify favorites): _____
_____ broiled or sautéed low-fat meats (chicken, turkey, veal, specify favorites): _____

From the healthy foods you already like, which you checked above, try to devise a number of diet meals that you'll find satisfying and pleasurable to eat. Some of the meals might include homemade soups and stews that take some time to prepare and can be done over the weekend. If you make a ritual out of cooking when you have time (turn on music to accompany you; work slowly and draw satisfaction from each step), you'll cut down feelings of food deprivation. But make sure you also devise some meals for the days when you're rushed. Use the recipes at the end of this chapter for inspiration. The low-fat cooking techniques and ingredients can be used to transform your own recipes into healthier eating.

If you're currently a heavy meat-and-potatoes-with-gravy eater, you probably need to acquire some new tastes, but it *can* be done! I used to despise plain low-fat yogurt, but one day a new brand came out that had none of the tartness of other versions, and yogurt was added to my favorite food list! So do experiment with low-fat foods. Take a slow trip through a large supermarket, browsing among the new products and reading labels. Food manufacturers are becoming more health-conscious, and you'll find lots of low-fat cheeses, sugar-free canned fruits and jams, and salt-reduced broths, soups, crackers, and even a light soy sauce.

A Personal Diet Plan

Now that you've identified the healthy foods you like, you can begin to plan menus based on them:

Leisurely Cooking Plan

List six healthy dishes, two for each meal, that you enjoy preparing when you have time.

Breakfast

1. _____
2. _____

Lunch

1. _____
2. _____

Dinner

1. _____
2. _____

Hurried Cooking Plan

List six healthy dishes, two for each meal, that you can prepare quickly (under 20 minutes) when you have little time to cook.

Breakfast

1. _____
2. _____

Lunch

1. _____
2. _____

Dinner

1. _____
2. _____

RECIPES

I consider myself a decent cook, though not a fancy one. I used to rely heavily on cookbooks, but since I began to eat healthfully I found it much more rewarding to be creative in the kitchen. Now I seldom cook the same dish the same way twice. I'm usually too busy to run out for a special ingredient called for by a recipe. Instead I use what's in the refrigerator, which I try to keep stocked with a variety of fresh vegetables, herbs, and fruits. In my cabinet, I always have pasta, brown rice, and more exotic grains such as couscous and bulgur wheat.

My knowledge of what ingredients are healthy and slimming and my feelings about what tastes I might enjoy at the moment determine how I spice and flavor my food. So I encourage you to use these recipes as inspiration and find your own ways to prepare the healthy foods that you particularly enjoy eating.

CURRIED CARROT SOUP

4 carrots, peeled and sliced
1 small Granny Smith apple, peeled, cored, and chopped
½ onion, chopped
3 cups chicken broth, with fat skimmed from top
1–2 teaspoons curry powder, to taste
¼ teaspoon cinnamon

Place the carrots, apple, onion, and chicken broth in a saucepan. Bring the liquid to a boil; reduce the heat and let it simmer until the carrots are tender, about 20 minutes.

Puree the mixture in a food processor or blender. Add the spices and serve, hot or chilled. *Serves 4.*

BROCCOLI SOUP

1 tablespoon corn or other vegetable oil
1 small onion, chopped
1 stalk celery, chopped
1 clove garlic, minced
³/₄ pound broccoli
4 cups chicken broth, with fat skimmed from top

In a saucepan, heat the oil and sauté the onion, celery, and garlic until soft. Separate the broccoli into flowerets and stems.

Add the chicken broth to the saucepan with the broccoli stems. Bring the liquid to a boil; reduce the heat, cover the pan, and simmer for 10 minutes. Add the broccoli flowerets and simmer another 5 to 7 minutes, until the broccoli is tender.

Puree the soup in a food processor or blender. *Serves 4, hot or cold.*

TABOULI

1 cup fine bulgur wheat (available in health food stores)
2 cups water
4 scallions, chopped
¹/₂ cup chopped fresh parsley
3 tablespoons chopped fresh mint, or 1¹/₂ teaspoons dried
2 tablespoons olive oil
3 tablespoons fresh lemon juice
2 tomatoes, chopped

In a saucepan, mix the bulgur with the water. Bring the water to a boil; reduce the heat and simmer until the water is absorbed and the bulgur tender, about 15 to 20 minutes. Let cool.

In a bowl, mix the bulgur with all the remaining ingredients except the tomatoes, and let sit for 30 minutes. Just before serving, stir in the tomatoes. *Serves 4.*

HUMMUS

2 cups cooked chick-peas
2 cloves garlic
2 tablespoons olive oil
1/2 cup fresh lemon juice
1/4 cup tahini (sesame paste—available in health food stores)
1/2 cup fresh parsley leaves

Mix all the ingredients in a food processor or blender and process until smooth. *Makes about 2 1/2 cups, about 4 servings.*

CHICKEN SALAD

3 boneless chicken breasts
1 1/2 cups broccoli flowerets
1 red pepper, seeded and chopped or sliced
4 scallions, chopped
2 tablespoons chopped walnuts

Dressing

3/4 cup low-fat yogurt
2 tablespoons chopped fresh dill, or 1 teaspoon dried
2 tablespoons fresh lemon juice
1 1/2 teaspoons Dijon mustard

Remove the skins from the chicken breasts. Add to a saucepan of water; bring the liquid to a boil, then reduce the heat and simmer for 15 minutes, or until the chicken is cooked through. Remove the chicken, cool, and cut into bite-size pieces.

In a saucepan, steam the broccoli until just tender. Rinse under cold water.

Add the chicken, broccoli, pepper, scallions, and walnuts to a bowl. In a small bowl, whisk together the dressing ingredients. Toss the dressing into the chicken salad and serve on a bed of lettuce. *Serves 4.*

PASTA SALAD

4 ounces fusilli or other shaped pasta
½ pound green beans, chopped into 1-inch pieces
2 cups broccoli flowerets
1 small yellow squash, sliced
½ red pepper, seeded and sliced
1 3-ounce can water-packed tuna, optional

Dressing

1 large clove garlic, minced
3 tablespoons chopped fresh basil or 2 teaspoons dried
Salt and pepper, to taste

Cook the pasta until it is just *al dente*. Rinse under cold water, drain, and let cool.

In a saucepan, steam the green beans, broccoli, and squash until just tender. Rinse under cold water, drain, and let cool.

Mix the pasta, beans, broccoli, squash, red pepper, and tuna (if using) in a bowl. Whisk together the dressing ingredients, pour over the pasta salad, and toss to mix thoroughly. *Serves 4.*

VEGETABLE ENCHILADAS

1 tablespoon corn oil
½ onion, chopped
½ red pepper, seeded and chopped
2 cups drained black beans, home-cooked or canned
2 tablespoons olive oil
2 tablespoons chopped fresh coriander, or 1 teaspoon dried
1 teaspoon cumin
8 corn tortillas
4 ounces part-skim cheese, such as mozzarella, shredded

In a saucepan, heat the oil and sauté the onion and red pepper in the corn oil until the vegetables are soft. Remove the pan from the heat and stir in the beans, olive oil, coriander, and cumin.

Soften the tortillas, one at a time, by quickly sautéing in a dry frying pan under a medium heat. After you heat each tortilla, lay it on a flat surface and spread some bean mixture down the middle. Roll up the tortilla and lay it in a lightly greased roasting pan. Repeat with the remaining tortillas and filling.

Spread the cheese over the tortillas and bake, at 350 degrees, for 20 to 30 minutes. Serve with salsa. *Serves 4.*

VEGETABLE LASAGNA

Sauce

1 tablespoon olive oil
1 onion, chopped
1/2 red pepper, seeded and chopped
2 cloves garlic, minced
1 15-ounce can crushed tomatoes
4 to 5 sun-dried tomatoes, optional
3 tablespoons chopped fresh basil or 1 1/2 teaspoons dried

1 tablespoon olive oil
2 zucchini, shredded
2 teaspoons grated lemon rind
Salt and pepper, to taste
1/2 pound lasagna
1 1/2 cups part-skim ricotta cheese
3 tablespoons Parmesan cheese
4 ounces part-skim mozzarella cheese, shredded

To make the sauce: In a saucepan, heat the oil and sauté the onion, red pepper, and garlic until the vegetables are soft. Add the remaining ingredients and simmer for 15 minutes.

While the sauce is simmering, cook the zucchini: In a skillet, heat 1 tablespoon olive oil and sauté the zucchini for 1 minute. Stir in the lemon rind and salt and pepper, remove from the heat, and reserve.

Cook the lasagna until it is *al dente*. (Meanwhile, preheat the oven to 350 degrees.) Rinse under cold water until it is cool enough to handle. Drain.

Spread a little sauce over the bottom of a flat casserole. Lay in 2 to 3 strips of lasagna. Spread the zucchini over the bottom layer, then cover it with another layer of lasagna. Spread ricotta and Parmesan on top and cover with the final layer of lasagna. Top the pasta with the sauce and sprinkle the mozzarella on top. Bake for 30 minutes or until the sauce is hot and bubbling. Let sit for 10 minutes before serving. *Serves 4.*

STIR-FRIED CHICKEN AND VEGETABLES

2 tablespoons peanut oil
2 chicken breasts, skinned, boned, and cut into 1½-inch chunks
½ pound asparagus, sliced diagonally
4 scallions, chopped
2 carrots, cut in julienne strips
1 yellow pepper, seeded and sliced
3 tablespoons chicken broth
2 tablespoons low-sodium soy sauce
1 tablespoon grated gingerroot

In a large skillet or wok, heat the oil and sauté the chicken quickly, stirring, until just tender. Remove the chicken. Add the vegetables to the oil and sauté, stirring, until they are just tender.

Return the chicken to the pan, stir in the chicken broth, soy sauce, and gingerroot. Let the broth come to a boil and cook another minute or two, while stirring. Serve over brown rice. *Serves 4.*

POACHED FRUIT DESSERT

Use your imagination in combining fresh and sugar-free frozen fruits. For example:

Combo 1

2 Cortland or Rome apples or ripe pears, peeled, cored, left whole
2 overripe bananas, cut in chunks
1 cup frozen strawberries
2 tablespoons orange or apple juice frozen concentrate
½ cup red wine

Combo 2

2 ripe pears, peeled, cored, sliced
2 Cortland or Rome apples, peeled, cored, sliced
1 tablespoon cinnamon
2 tablespoons orange or apple juice frozen concentrate
1 tablespoon fruit-flavored liqueur (optional)

Topping (optional)

2 tablespoons plain low-fat yogurt
Cinnamon to taste

Microwave: Combine all ingredients in microwave-safe casserole with cover, or cover with microwave-safe plastic wrap. Microwave on high for 6 minutes. Remove cover carefully and baste fruit with juice in pan. Microwave for 12 minutes for whole fruits, 5 for sliced fruits.

Stovetop: Add water to increase liquids to 2 cups. Combine all ingredients in saucepan with lid. Simmer very slowly for 20 minutes or until tender, basting frequently and adding liquid if needed, until fruit is tender.

Top with yogurt sprinkled with cinnamon, if desired. *Serves 2–3.*

PART 5

THE HEALTHY WALKER

12

Pampering Your Feet

It's not unusual to come back from an especially long walk and find that your feet are aching a bit. There's no reason to be alarmed. Simply give your feet the warming and massage treatment described in this chapter and they'll soon be ready for more high stepping.

Sometimes, however, the problem persists. An area on your foot is red, hot, and swollen. Or you get a stabbing pain in your heel as you walk. Or your shins and ankles ache for hours. Beginning walkers often think that walking causes these problems. But as this chapter will show you, it's usually not the exercise but how your foot is rubbing inside your shoe or an inherited arch or toe problem that is causing the problem. Some of these foot problems require medical care. Often a comfortable, custom-fitted shoe insert, called an orthotic, can turn problem feet into happy ones. For more minor problems, this chapter includes some of my personal recipes for cooking up happier feet.

Whatever the cause, if your feet hurt, do something for them. We expect our feet to step quickly over miles of pavement or dirt while we're walking. So we should do something in return—at least on occasion.

Post-Walking Foot Aches

Feet have muscles too. As you work into the Walk It Off! program you're most likely going to be using those foot muscles a lot more than you did before. So don't be surprised if they ache a little after your walk. On occasion, you may even have cramps in your legs.

> *Footprints in the sand* are a good way to check how your feet turn out as you walk. They should turn outward only the tiniest bit, perhaps an inch or two. If your toes turn out more than a couple of inches, or turn inward, see a podiatrist about corrective measures.

I find that my feet never bother me when I'm actually walking. But as soon as I get home and take off my walking shoes, they start complaining. Usually a 5-minute rest with my feet up resolves the problem. But the very best treatment is a foot massage. I often use this as my "me break" to reward myself for walking. That means I take special care to make the experience pleasurable by turning on some soft music, using perfumed lotions, and reveling in the time devoted to myself.

Whatever the cause of your foot pain, and even if you have no pain at all, a massage is something you can do to make your feet feel good. It relaxes the muscles, stimulates circulation, and gives instant relief to tired, sweaty, swollen, itching, or blistered feet.

A thorough foot massage has three parts. First, there's the "warm-up"—applying heat and/or moisture to the feet for at least 10 minutes to soften and relax them. Then there's the massage itself, a deep squeezing and kneading of the muscles in the feet. Lastly, there's the foot refresher—applying lotion, powder, and perhaps toenail polish to pretty up your feet.

Warm-up

There are a number of methods you can use for heating and softening your feet:

- Sit on the edge of the bathtub with your feet under the faucet for about 10 minutes. Turn on the water to a warm temperature, and slowly increase the temperature until it's as hot as you can tolerate; then gradually decrease to a cool finish. Your feet will feel tingly and fresh.
- Create a foot tub from a large tub or pot. Fill with warm water and Epsom salts. Soak for 15 minutes.
- Wrap feet in hot, moist, thin towels. Use a dry one next to your skin, then wrap that in a towel soaked in very hot water. Repeat two or three layers, ending with a dry towel to keep the heat in. Then sit for 15 to 20 minutes and let the heat do its job.
- Use a heating pad to warm feet. But if your feet are very cold to begin with after a winter walk, wait until they warm up to room temperature to avoid burns.
- Buy a commercial footbath that bathes and massages feet. Automatic controls allow you to adjust heat and speed on the tiny vibrating massage fingers to comfortable levels.

Massage

Once your feet are warm and relaxed, sit with one leg crossed over the other with the bottom of the sole of one foot facing you. You may want to use a little moisturizing or body lotion to keep your foot lubricated as you work.

Using your thumbs, massage the foot in deep, circular motions, concentrating on very small areas. If you find an area that is knotted up, knead until the knot caused by tense muscles diminishes and disappears. Slap the sole of your foot lightly with a relaxed wrist.

After you've worked the entire bottom of the sole, turn your foot and massage the top of the foot with your thumbs. Work more gently on this softer skin, stroking outward to stretch the tendons. Again, work on a small area at a time and cover the whole top of the foot.

Then work the toes. Grasp each between thumb and forefinger and give it a good tug. Wiggle the toe from side to side. Then switch feet!

When you've massaged both feet, you may want to clip your toenails and apply some kind of treat. Moisturizer or skin cream can be applied first, to further soften the skin. Then after-shave or a facial astringent makes a refreshing splash. Talcum powder feels good and makes a nice finish. Women may find this a good moment to apply toenail polish.

Bumps, Lumps, and Swellings

Some types of foot pain can't be resolved with a simple massage. Here is a rundown of the foot problems walkers complain about most, and some home remedies for dealing with them.

Blisters

This very common problem among walkers usually occurs because of a too-new, too-tight, or improperly fitting shoe. Blisters result from friction—the rubbing of the skin against a hard edge of a shoe. The blister is the body's defense against the shearing force of the shoe moving against the foot. Most blisters start off with redness, some swelling, and a burning sensation. Sometimes the entire foot feels hot.

If you feel a blister starting to develop, care for it immediately. If caught in time, the red area may not develop into the characteristic blister filled with pus. Begin your home treatment with a very gentle foot massage; then cover the area with a bandage or other protection. Check the fit of your shoes. If they're new and not yet broken in, wearing a bandage for a few days over the reddened area may prevent blisters and give the shoes a chance to soften. It's also important to wear socks that fit well. Some shoe stores now carry "walker's socks," which feature extra padding for blister-prone areas.

If you have bony toes, you might keep a moleskin over sensitive areas. Moleskin is pinkish, feltlike foot padding that can be purchased in any drugstore. Many athletes and dancers put lamb's wool over the tops of their toes to prevent blisters. Petroleum jelly (Vaseline) and foot powders also help reduce friction.

If a blister does form, here's how to deal with it:

- Cleanse skin with alcohol or an iodine solution.
- Sterilize a pocketknife or needle by holding it in a flame for 60 seconds.
- Puncture the blister, but leave the top part in place to serve as a cover and avoid infection.
- Apply a topical antibiotic cream (Neosporin, Bacitracin, Polysporin).
- Cover with a bandage or a sterile piece of gauze and tape.

Calluses

The callus is the number-one foot problem for walkers. It's a buildup of dead, thickened, yellowish skin in an area where excess pressure or friction occurs. Calluses usually occur on the bottom of the foot or along the outside of the big toe. The body produces a callus to cushion the underlying tender skin from pressure at points where the foot has little fat or natural padding.

Unless a callus bothers you, there's no harm in just ignoring it. I admit I do remove mine once or twice a year, using the "recipe" below. The reason I do it is to save money on stockings! Rough, callused skin can cut right through the soles of panty hose.

Some calluses need to be removed because they are quite painful and can make walking a chore. Painful calluses are most likely to be found on the balls of the feet and may be caused by abnormal motion in your forefoot. People with low-arched feet are particularly prone to this problem. If you have painful callus buildup under the ball behind your big toe, however, you probably have a high-arched foot with a biomechanical problem.

Sometimes a callus that has been pain-free suddenly starts to hurt. The skin has thickened so much that it causes constant irritation to the softer surrounding tissues. The spot may become red, puffy, and very tender. You may also feel a burning sensation, especially if you've been taking your walks on hard pavements.

Some commercially available callus cream and ointments will eliminate skin buildup, but they do it with salicylic acid, a very caustic ingredient that can harm the surrounding skin. So use these with caution. I prefer to give my patients my own recipe for a less dangerous callus remover:

- Crush five or six aspirin tablets to a powder.
- Mix with 1 tablespoon of lemon juice and 1 tablespoon of water.
- Apply paste to all the hard-skin spots on your foot.
- Put your entire foot in a plastic bag.
- Wrap a warm towel around the plastic.
- Leave on for 10 minutes so the paste can penetrate the skin.
- Unwrap your foot and scrub the dead skin away with pumice stone (a rough-edged stone that can be purchased in drugstores).

If this treatment doesn't work, see a podiatrist, who will soften the calluses and then use a surgical blade to pare them away. But please don't try to cut calluses away yourself! It's easy to go too deep and cut into live tissue, which really hurts. I've had to treat too many self-administered wounds to want any walker to take this chance.

A podiatrist will be able to help correct any physical problem, such as misaligned bone or a crooked toe, that is causing the callus buildup. He or she can prescribe an orthotic—a custom-made shoe insert that redistributes your weight inside your shoe and corrects the bony abnormalities that cause calluses and foot pain.

Corns

A corn looks like its name—it's a round yellow area of thick skin in the shape of a corn kernel. Like calluses, corns are your body's response to friction and pressure. Most corns occur between the fourth and fifth little toes. If you develop one, you should immediately go out and buy a pair of shoes that fit more comfortably and don't crush your toes together. You may have to buy a larger size or a different style of shoe to allow your toes to lie flat.

Corn pain may come from a bursa—a fluid-filled sac between the corn and the bone that becomes inflamed and enlarged. Shrinking the bursal sac and taking pressure off nearby nerves can bring temporary pain relief. Here's how to do it:

- Mix Epsom salts (purchase in a drugstore) and warm water in a foot pan or bathtub.
- Soak your foot until the pain stops.
- Apply moisturizing cream.
- Cover the corn area in plastic for at least 15 minutes.
- Unwrap the foot and rub with pumice stone in a side-to-side motion to remove hard corn skin.
- Wear open-toed sandals, or protect the corn with a piece of moleskin until it has completely disappeared.

Ingrown Toenails

The wrong walking shoes can aggravate and contribute to ingrown toenails. They occur when the side of a toenail (most often on the big toe) cuts into the skin around the nail. The area can become very sensitive to pressure, especially from the side of the shoe.

If you feel pressure or notice inflammation around a toenail, try this home remedy:

- Wear toeless sandals or shoes that do not press on the toe.
- If an infection is present, soak the foot in iodine solution to reduce inflammation.
- Trim nails and clean cuticle area.
- Apply antibiotic cream.

If pain persists, do yourself a favor and see a podiatrist or physician. He or she can remove the part of the nail that curves in and causes your problem.

Bunions

A hereditary imbalance in the muscles of the feet is usually the root cause of bunions. The imbalance causes the arch to sag and the ligaments to stretch, leading to a deviation, or leaning, of the big toe. The big toe is no longer straight, and it twists toward the second toe. This causes a bony protrusion on the outside of the big toe that may be pronounced enough to be noticeable through a shoe. This occurs more frequently in women, who have a lighter and more easily injured bone structure. Although I've seen some cases of juvenile bunions, it mostly occurs with aging. Shoes may contribute to bunions, but they are never the only cause. People who live on tropical islands and never wear shoes also get them!

Bunions that don't hurt should not interfere with a walking program. Painful bunions are accompanied by bursitis, an inflammation of the bursal sac beneath and next to the bone. You know you have bursitis if a whitish area appears when you push down on the bump; this area turns red when you stop pressing on it.

Painful bunions require professional help. But if you've got an inflamed one on a Saturday night, here's a home treatment:

- Apply an ice pack to the bunion for 15 minutes, three or four times a day, to reduce acute inflammation.
- Mix 1 cup vinegar into 1 gallon of warm water and soak area for 15 minutes to alleviate pain.
- Reduce pressure to the area by wearing a very wide shoe, sandal, or sneaker with a hole cut out.
- Take aspirin for pain.
- Create your own bunion pad by cutting moleskin or foam rubber in a doughnut shape.

Only surgery can eliminate bunions, and it's something serious walkers should consider. A podiatrist will discuss your options. Many of my patients tell me they're very glad they decided on surgery to correct the underlying muscle alignment and eliminate the bunion. It's a relatively small price to pay for the freedom to walk without pain.

Heel Pain

There are two major causes of pain in the heels. One is callus buildup at the back of the foot that gets so dried out that a fissure or crack develops in the heel. Psoriasis, fungal infections, and overweight can also contribute to cracked heels. A cracked heel can make walking painful and invite infections.

With certain precautions, a cracked heel does not have to interfere with your walking program. Follow the treatment for removing calluses and rub with a pumice stone until you eliminate the callus buildup. Continue to lubricate the skin of the feet at least three times a week with moisturizer as a regular preventive practice.

Spurs are another cause of heel pain. A spur is a bony protrusion on the bottom of the foot, visible on X-ray, that is caused by a growth of calcium that has begun to project downward. If the calcium spur touches your plantar fascia—the thick piece of tissue underneath the skin on the sole of your foot—it can be quite painful. The pain you feel is the tissue being torn by the bony protrusion.

If you feel pain in your heel as soon as you get up in the morning and touch your feet on the ground, you probably have a heel spur. Heel spur pain is always greatest after rest. That's because as you walk after a rest, you're stressing your foot tissue and tearing it anew with the heel spur.

To keep a heel spur from interfering with your walking program, it pays to buy a pair of walking shoes with extra padding under the arch. The firm arch will take some of the pressure off your heel. You can also buy extra arch padding and insert it into your walking shoe.

If the heel spur becomes inflamed because of a fluid-filled bursal sac, it may make your whole leg ache. For immediate pain relief, take an analgesic (aspirin, acetaminophen, ibuprofen) and elevate the foot and apply ice to the heel for 20 minutes. Then try putting a foam or felt heel pad in your shoe (available in many shoe stores). If this doesn't help, you can get a special orthotic made to fit your heel. Ultrasound pain therapy, special footbaths, and surgery are sometimes needed.

Sole Pain

The older you get, the thinner the fat pads on the bottom of your feet become. The less fat you have, the hotter your feet get from the friction. A pair of orthotics can substitute for the lost fat pads and relieve intermittent pain.

If the burning sensation occurs when you wear a particular pair of shoes, either get rid of them or ask a shoe repair shop to insert a new permanent innersole of leather or another natural lining.

"Walking is not for sissies."—Steve Reeves, former Mr. Universe, who began walking after a series of jogging injuries

If the bottoms of your feet burn only after you walk long distances, you may have a gait problem and should be checked by a doctor. If you have constant (rather than occasional) burning on both soles that is not caused by a new pair of shoes, you should seek prompt medical attention. Medications, alcohol, chemical poisoning, anemia, or diabetes may be the cause of the problem.

Aching Arches

If you haven't walked much and suddenly start a walking program, aching arches may result simply from using previously underused muscles. Pain in this area can also occur on days that you do a lot of extra standing or climbing steps. A good foot massage and rest and a gradually increasing exercise program should resolve the problem.

Runners and walkers sometimes develop tendinitis—inflammation of the small tendons that attach the muscles in your feet to the bones. Rest and ice followed by heat is the best way to treat tendinitis. Wrapping an elastic bandage around the area for support and buying a pair of shoes with extra arch support should help. If you have tried the home remedies and your arches still ache, see a podiatrist or orthopedist. You may need an orthotic.

Sometimes starting a walking program calls attention to a previously ignored arch problem. A healthy arch springs back into shape with each step you take. If your arch sinks too low and touches the ground with each step, you have a fallen arch or flat feet, which can making walking quite painful. Consult a physician before you continue with the walking program.

Ankle Pain

If your ankle hurts—whether or not you remember twisting it—you may have a strain or a sprain. Strain is caused by overstretching muscles, tendons, or ligaments; a sprain is an actual tearing of these tissues. If you're overweight, pregnant, or double-jointed, you may be prone to sprained ankles. Certain sports—ice skating, tennis, and racquetball, for example—also stress the ankles. Pregnancy and obesity put stress on the ankles via increased weight. In pregnancy, certain hormones also create relaxation in the ligaments, which makes them prone to sprains.

If you hear a "pop" when you bang or turn your ankle, you know that you have torn tissue. Prolonged pain, swelling, and bruising are other signs that you need an immediate X-ray and medical attention.

The prescription for a twisted ankle can be found in the acronym RICE: Rest, Ice, Compression, and Exercise. Rest the ankle completely for 24 to 48 hours; apply ice packs on and off until swelling disappears; compress by wrapping an elastic bandage around the ankle; and exercise by gently stretching and rotating the foot to increase range of motion.

Shin Pain

When I started a jogging program after years of sedentary life, I found myself with swollen, painful shins, a condition diagnosed as shin splints. Shin splints are much less common in walkers, but they do sometimes occur and are particularly painful in walkers who go up and down hills. Aerobic dance on very hard surfaces can also cause shin splints, as can exercising without stretching heel cords. (The toe-tapping exercise in Chapter 3 is an easy way to keep heel cords limber and injury-free.)

A shin splint occurs when the two muscles attached to your shin have pulled away from the bone. The symptoms are a leg that feels tight and perhaps swollen and hurts when you walk. You may have spots of inflammation on your lower leg.

Treatment:

- Put ice packs on the inflamed muscles at the site of pain.
- Rest for 24 to 48 hours.
- Stretch muscles by flexing your feet slowly up and down before walking.
- Wrap your leg in an elastic bandage if that helps relieve pain.
- Use analgesics as needed.
- If the pain doesn't go away in a day or two, see a doctor for an X-ray. You may have a stress fracture.

If your feet hurt, you're not likely to draw much pleasure from walking. In my podiatry practice I see many people who have had foot pain for years. They finally decide to do something about it when they begin a walking program. Most foot pain is curable—usually by treatment no more drastic than cutting away a corn or prescribing a shoe insert. So don't let foot problems interfere with your walking. See your doctor and get back on the road!

13

Questions and Answers About Walking and Health

As a nation, we're beginning to understand that there's relatively little medical science can do about our major health problems—heart disease, cancer, arthritis, and other chronic conditions—once they occur. But there's a lot we can do to help prevent these problems from disrupting our lives to begin with.

Regular walking, a low-fat diet, and abstention from nicotine are the trio of health measures recommended for the prevention of virtually all chronic conditions. They also help combat many of the health problems we used to think were a natural part of the aging process, such as bone loss and skeletal shrinking, a shuffling, hestitant gait, and lack of energy.

When I speak to corporate groups about walking, I'm asked many questions about the specific ways walking affects various body systems and diseases. Here are some of the more commonly asked questions, along with the answers I've culled from both my own medical training and my research into walking and health.

Can walking help me to stop smoking?

Nicotine is one of the hardest addictions to break. Yet it's really worth the trouble, since, as you no doubt know, smoking is one of the most damaging things you can do to your body.

One reason nicotine is hard to give up is that it increases the production of adrenaline in the body, which stimulates the heart to work harder. A quickened pulse rate, higher blood pressure, and the pumping of more blood to the brain makes people feel more alive and mentally active. That's a nice feeling, and one that smokers are loath to give up. People who stop smoking often feel tired, sluggish, and unmotivated.

The good news is that even a short walk of a quarter of a mile produces the same positive physiological result as smoking. The longer, aerobic walks of the Walk It Off! program are natural energizers, gearing up the body's blood circulation and metabolic rates. Physicians and patients report that walking makes it easier to quit smoking because it reduces the craving for the nicotine high.

I started the Walk It Off! program a few weeks ago. Now I'm feeling pain in my lower back. Could walking be the cause?

Anyone with back pain that lasts more than a few days should see a doctor to make sure there is no disease process, such as a vascular disorder, a tumor, a kidney ailment, or a neurological problem. Most of the time, however, pain in the lower back is due not to any disease but to the way you're standing, walking, and using your feet.

If back pain begins after you start walking regularly, you should be checked for foot problems. If your arch is too high, the foot's ability to absorb shocks is lessened, and the shock of each step you take is sent straight up your leg to your spine. A flat, or pronated, arch can also cause back pain by throwing you off balance and putting extra pressure on the muscles of the lower back. Often an orthotic insert designed for your foot and worn inside your walking shoes can resolve the problem and allow you to continue exercising without pain.

If the back pain has come from strain or a degenerated disk, walking and some special back exercises may be exactly what you need to help relieve it. This was discovered by a University of Miami neurosurgeon who prescribed walking in order to get his back-surgery patients in better shape before the operation. He found, to his surprise, that walking worked so well that many patients didn't need the surgery! So do trace down the origins—and don't use the back pain as an excuse to stay inactive!

Can walking relieve constipation?

Walking can be the best laxative there is. It works like a fiber-rich diet, speeding up sluggish digestion and keeping bowels regular, thus preventing constipation. For best results, combine your walking program with a diet that emphasizes fruits, vegetables, and whole grains.

I have frequent asthma attacks. Is it safe for me to start a walking program?

For many years children and adults with asthma were advised not to exercise for fear that it would trigger an attack. But recently a number of world-class athletes who have asthma—such as Danny Manning, the 1987–88 NCAA College Basketball Player of the Year—have led a turnaround in thinking.

Even if they have no intention of going for the gold, exercise can improve the lung function of people with asthma, as studies by Dr. François Hass, a pulmonary physiologist at New York University Hospital, have shown.

Exercise-induced asthma attacks affect an estimated 12 to 15 percent of the population, according to the American Academy of Allergy and Immunology. If you have a history of asthma, ask your doctor about what precautions you should take before embarking on the Walk It Off! program. Carrying an inhaler and taking daily preventive medications may be advisable. When the air is cool, cold, or dry, wearing a scarf or mask around the nose and mouth to help warm and moisten incoming air is another tested way to avoid asthma attacks.

A walking program undertaken under medical supervision is a great way for people with asthma to build lung capacity, fitness, and self-confidence.

Can walking really help me live longer?

"If new studies are to believed, every hour you walk may add another hour to your life." That was the pitch *Vogue* magazine used to get readers walking. Personally, I think that's oversell. How long an individual lives is affected by many factors aside from how much exercise he or she gets.

However, walking does increase your chances of living a longer, healthier life. A study of Harvard University alumni found that the risk of early death was lower for those who expended more calories on physical activity. If you walk 2 miles a day, you may reduce your risk of death by 27 percent compared to a sedentary person.

Osteoporosis runs in my family. Can walking help prevent it?

Osteoporosis means "porous" bones. On X-ray, the bone is not solid but looks like a honeycomb or Swiss cheese. On the outside, we see a dowager's hump, a shrinking of the body, and brittle bones that are prone to fractures.

Hormones, diet, and exercise—as well as your genes—help determine whether you'll get this progressive thinning of the bones that affects many postmenopausal women. Walking can help your bones maintain and even gain strength and density. When you walk, as much as 400 pounds of force travels up your legs and spine with each step. The force of gravity, as well as your own effort, causes your muscles to pull on your bones and stimulate the bone to take in more strengthening calcium.

Although our bones tend to lose strength as we age, regular walking can slow down and even reverse this trend. In a study at

Tufts University, for example, postmenopausal women walked briskly 45 minutes a day, four days a week, for a year. At the year's end the bone density in the lower spine had increased by 3 percent. An inactive group of women of similar age had an average bone *loss* of 10 percent during the year. "From what we see, exercise may be one of the *best* ways to stop or prevent age-related bone loss," says William Evans, Ph.D., chief of the Tufts University laboratory. A National Institutes of Health consensus panel agreed and recommended a program of modest weight-bearing exercise to help prevent osteoporosis. Walking is especially important for women whose mothers or grandmothers have osteoporosis.

Medications and summer walking may not mix. Certain prescription drugs (including sedatives and certain heart medications) can dangerously interfere with sweating. Check with your doctor.

I've recently had a heart attack. My doctor recommended that I start a walking program, but I'm nervous about overdoing it. What do you recommend?

Not too long ago, many physicians believed that vigorous physical exercise might contribute to atherosclerosis, the cause of heart attacks. Heart attack survivors were advised to refrain from any physical activity. However, since the 1950s a number of major scientific studies have shown that regular exercise can prevent recurrent heart attacks.

Studies have also shown that people who exercise regularly tend to recover more quickly and completely after a heart attack or coronary bypass surgery. Walking is a favored exercise, since it carries much less risk of temporarily overloading the heart and provoking sudden death than more intense regimes.

I suggest that you not try to "go it alone" with walking, but seek out a postcardiac rehabilitation program at your local hospital,

Y, or community center. Professional supervision and group support will help you learn to exercise within your limits and gain confidence.

Perhaps the worse aftereffect of having a heart attack is the fear of having another one. A regular, supervised walking program is one of the best ways you can begin to set aside this fear.

I'm pregnant. Is it okay for me to walk?

Because it is low-impact and can be adjusted to almost any level of fitness, brisk walking is an excellent exercise for pregnant women. It has been found safe for both the mother and the unborn child, according to an article in the *Journal of the American Medical Association*. After the birth, walking helps restore muscle tone and body weight to prepregnancy levels. But, since every pregnancy is different, I urge you ask your obstetrician for advice before plunging in.

During the later months of pregnancy, certain safety precautions are advisable. The body produces hormones that relax the ligaments and allow the pelvic region to expand to permit the birth; this relaxation also makes the ligaments prone to sprains. The extra weight of pregnancy also puts a strain on the legs and feet and can throw a woman off balance. So be especially careful that your walking shoes provide maximum stability. I also recommend walking only on smooth, level surfaces, such as a track.

Can walking help control diabetes?

About 80 percent of people with adult-onset diabetes are overweight. Taking off the extra pounds, with the help of walking, is a great aid to controlling the disease. Walking also helps by increasing the uptake of blood sugar (glucose) by the muscles and may increase sensitivity to insulin. A combination of weight loss and regular exercise can make it much easier for diabetics to keep their blood sugar under control and feel well.

It's important for people with diabetes to consult their doctors before starting to walk. A stress test may be recommended before starting any exercise program. Those with diabetes should also learn to take especially good care of their feet. Diabetes sufferers who develop nerve damage in their lower legs are in danger of not feeling an injury when it occurs; even minor blisters and cuts can turn into major problems if they become infected. Because circulation, particularly in the feet, tends to be poor in diabetics, it's harder for them to fight infection.

I'm in my late 60s. What should my target heart rate be?

"In our aging population, strength, flexibility, and balance are probably going to be much more important than measurements of cardiovascular fitness," said Dr. Ronald LaPorte of the University of Pittsburgh at a round table on the health benefits of exercise in *The Physician and Sportsmedicine*. Strength, flexibility, and balance are the critical elements in preventing falls and making it easier to perform the routine activities of life. "I think that being able to lift, reach, and climb stairs is potentially more important than the level of cardiovascular fitness," said Dr. LaPorte.

"I have two doctors, my left leg and my right leg."—JOHN MA-
CAULAY TREVELYAN, English historian, who lived to be 86.

Walking is the ideal exercise for older people, because it not only gives their heart and lungs a workout, but it strengthens muscles throughout the body, keeps them limber, and improves posture and balance. So my advice to older exercisers is not to worry too much about pulse rates. Make sure you don't walk too fast by checking now and then that you can speak comfortably and don't feel out of breath. Challenge yourself by making sure you walk at least 20 minutes four or five times a week. You'll not only stay healthier longer, but the lilt in your step will make you feel and look younger.

I live in a very warm climate. Can walking in hot weather cause heatstroke?

When the temperature and humidity soar, any kind of exertion can cause heat injury. The best prevention is to walk in the early morning or at dusk when the temperature cools, or to find an indoor, air-conditioned place to walk.

Everyone who walks in warm weather should know the warning signs of heat injury. Heat cramps are painful muscle spasms, usually in the legs or abdomen, that occur after exercise. Heavy sweating; headache; weak, rapid pulse; dilated pupils; and cold, clammy, pale skin are the symptoms of heat exhaustion. These conditions should be treated by removing the person to a cool area, out of the sun, loosening clothing, giving a sip of cold water, and massaging cramped areas.

The more serious symptoms of heatstroke can be fatal and need emergency medical attention. They are rapid pulse; hot, dry skin; lack of sweating; headache; dizziness; delirium; loss of consciousness; and high body temperature. The victim should be moved to a cool area and covered with ice packs until medical treatment arrives.

What are the advantages of walking vs. running?

Several studies have shown that people who do strenuous exercises, such as running, are subject to a high rate of injuries. They often drop out. When it comes to reaping the health benefits from exercise, a little exercise, done consistently over a lifetime, is what counts most, even more than the intensity of the exercise done.

Is it really true that a walking program can help me look younger?

I've seen a number of people turn back the clock and get results from walking that surpass many an expensive, painful face-lift. Many of the things we associate with aging are actually due to inactivity. A sedentary life allows your body to start dismantling itself. Your ability to use oxygen, pump blood, produce red blood cells, create new bone, assimilate glucose, and expel waste begins to decline rapidly in the middle years if your life is spent sitting. This biological decline is mirrored in how you look and feel. Your skin starts to sag, your eyes dull, you gain weight, you feel weak and lethargic, your step becomes hesitant. In short, you look old. This can occur as early as age 30!

The Walk It Off! program can put the pep back in your step and the glint back in your eye. Your skin will take on a youthful glow. And as your mood improves, you'll feel younger . . . which is more than half the battle.

I have arthritis that is sometimes very painful. Is it realistic for me to expect to walk?

Doctors once advised arthritic patients against exercising, but now, according to the American Arthritis Association, more and more are encouraging walking. Walking helps to strengthen the muscles around the joints, which may prevent joint injury and disfigurement. It also seems to relieve some of the pain that occurs when bones rub together.

Walking is also a natural mood elevator, which can fight the vicious circle of pain leading to depression. Sitting and feeling stiff may hurt more than moving.

I advise people with painful arthritis to begin walking very slowly. Walk only as far as you can without feeling more pain than you had when you started. If that means you only walk across the room, fine. One or two blocks, fine. If you can go farther, but are afraid pain will flare up and leave you stranded far from home, don't go on long-distance walks. Walk around and around the block where you live.

Increase your time and distance very slowly, perhaps 10 percent every two weeks. Work with your physician. You may need strengthening and stretching exercises as well.

Many arthritic people find that walking in water (see Chapter 9) is the most comfortable exercise. The water is soothing and displaces body weight, putting less stress on the joints. The Arthritis Foundation and the YMCA cosponsor water exercise programs.

Does walking really prevent cancer?

Scientists are just beginning to answer this question. In a ground-breaking study, researchers at Kuakini Medical Center in Honolulu found that increased activity significantly reduced the risk of colon cancer in a twenty-one-year study of over 8,000 Hawaiian/Japanese men. Large Swedish and California studies both found higher risk of cancer of the colon for men in sedentary occupations (such as accounting, bookkeeping, law, and music) than those in active jobs (carpentry, gardening, mail carrying, plumbing). The anticancer effect may have something to do with digestion and bowel habits.

An ongoing study by Harvard's Dr. Rose Frisch found that women with active life-styles from their youth had lower risks of developing cancer of the breast and the reproductive organs. It's not yet clear what type or level of physical activity is needed to get an anticancer effect, but walking sure can't hurt.

I have high blood pressure. Can walking help me get off medication?

Exercise can help bring down your blood pressure, but it isn't the whole answer. Stopping smoking, losing weight, and eating a low-fat diet are also very important. If you have only mild high blood pressure, moderate exercise may be as effective as hypertensive medications in lowering it. In general, though, regular exercise doesn't normalize high blood pressure, though it may lower it a bit.

Don't make the common mistake of thinking you can safely stop taking these medicines just because you've started walking. High blood pressure raises the risks of coronary heart disease, stroke, and kidney disease. Blood pressure can rebound dangerously if you suddenly stop taking prescribed medications. Instead, talk to your doctor about your walking and see if it's feasible for your medications to be gradually reduced. Walking also aids long-term weight loss and control, which indirectly lowers blood pressure. And walking may prevent the development of high blood pressure.

Good news for walkers: A study at Rutgers University found that moderate- or low-intensity exercise (like walking) is better than high-intensity exercise (like running, or aerobic dance) for lowering blood pressure.

I like to walk in the winter, but my feet and hands often feel tingly and tender when I come home. Is this a sign of frostbite?

If sensation in your hands and feet quickly returns to normal after they've warmed to room temperature, your skin has gotten chilled, but not frostbitten. Even so, you should double up on your skin protection. You can wear a pair of wool socks under a pair of mittens for extra warmth. And try two of three layers of socks— provided you own or can buy a pair of walking shoes that are roomy enough to allow for the extra bulk.

Signs of frostbite include pain, numbness, and eventual loss of function in the affected area. Careful rewarming can prevent permanent damage. Don't place frostbitten or chilled skin under very hot running water or a heating pad. Your sensations have gone numb and you might burn your skin without realizing it. Instead, rewarm gradually by careful soaking in lukewarm water.

Does walking affect cholesterol levels?

Although it's long been known that exercise reduces the risk of heart disease, scientists have thought that it did so by reducing weight and thus the levels of fats in the bloodstream. But a study by Rockefeller University scientists recently found that even when weight levels are constant, exercise reduces the levels of dangerous fats in the bloodstreams.

Exercise doesn't lower the total levels of artery-clogging cholesterol in the blood. To do that you need to eat less saturated fat and cholesterol and fewer total calories. But walking can help increase the ratio of good fat (high-density lipid or HDL) to bad fat (low-density lipid or LDL) in your blood. It's the LDL that lines the arteries and causes hardening or atherosclerosis. HDL helps rid the bloodstream of excess cholesterol, taking it to the liver, where it can be excreted.

Exercise, combined with weight loss, can increase your HDL level. It's the distance covered, not the speed, that really counts, so walkers do as well as joggers. Some studies suggest that an activity threshold of as little as 10 miles a week can make a difference in HDL levels.

I am 81 years old. My doctor said it was safe for me to walk, but I find myself getting tired very quickly. What do you recommend?

Elderly people, and those who have been ill recently, can begin by walking 1 or 2 minutes, resting for 1 minute, and then repeating this cycle until they feel tired. That's the recommendation of the President's Council on Sports and Fitness. Even if you can walk in this manner only for 5 or 10 minutes at the beginning, it pays to persist. As the President's Council points out, where you start is not important. It's where you're going that counts!

Is 20 minutes a day really enough exercise to improve my health?

Amazingly, yes! You may want to do more, and the Walk It Off! program encourages you to very gradually work your way up to 60-minute walks, four times a week. But even if the only change you make is to go from no exercise to 20-minute walks three or four times a week, you're doing yourself a lot of good. Keep it up, consistently, for the rest of your life, and you're not only likely to live longer and suffer less disease, you'll have the strength, energy, and good mood to enjoy your healthy old age!

PART

6

ADVANCED WALKING

Fitness has a way of sneaking up on the regular walker. When I first started walking I wasn't very concerned with my heart rate or muscle strength. I was interested in losing weight and feeling good. But little by little I began to notice I was actually becoming physically fit. For the first 18 months of my walking program, my heart rate didn't increase very much until toward the end of my walk. But as I approached my second year of walking, I began to notice that I felt warm, even sweaty, after just 10 minutes out. I got that glorious sense of "shifting gears" that occurs when your heart rate speeds up and the resultant extra blood circulation gives you a fresh spurt of energy. Once I shift into that higher gear, walking becomes easier, even effortless, and I start looking for hills or staircases to increase the challenge.

I also began to notice that my muscles were getting stronger. It was less of a problem to carry heavy grocery bags. My legs felt less tired, even after standing for hours doing surgery. And perhaps most exciting, when my husband and I went out for the evening, I became an inexhaustible dancer. I could rock for hours and feel sorry when the band took a break.

For the first time in my life I felt the wonderful sense of power that comes with feeling physically strong. When summertime rolled around, I found myself looking forward to playing tennis, a game I used to play only with great reluctance. Before I became a walker, I limited my tennis to doubles matches, which take far less energy than singles, since you don't have to run across the court after the tennis ball. But after two years of walking I became an avid singles player, sometimes lasting up to three hours on the court.

Another sign of how much walking had changed my life became evident when I took a trip to the Alaska wilderness in 1986. It included numerous hikes in the Mount McKinley region. Many members of the group tour experienced extreme exhaustion and decided to sit out some of the more strenuous climbs. But, to my amazement, I found myself at the head of the hiking group. I could keep up with tour guides who had trekked the same mountains on many occasions. And all from just four or five walking sessions, from 20 to 60 minutes each, a week! I don't look like a physically powerful person, and my friends were amazed at my stamina and lack of fatigue. I can remember sitting at the top of the mountain enjoying a light snack while other members of the group were still far below, huffing and puffing their way up. What a great feeling for a girl who had always been chosen last for school sports teams!

This final section of *Walk It Off!* is dedicated to the advanced walker—the one who has made walking a regular habit and is beginning to reap the mental and physical rewards. This stage has some perils as well. It's easy, now, to become bored with walking, to take it for granted, to get restless with the routine. And there's always a danger that unexpected changes in your life can interrupt your walking routine and create lapses or relapses. In these chapters I hope to show you how to combat boredom creatively and maintain your hard-won walking habit for a lifetime.

14

Games People Play While Walking

When you first begin to walk, there's plenty of challenge just in getting out there—making yourself do it, carving a time and place for walking in your life. But after two months, three months, a year, of regular walking, this does become easier. You have the walking habit. You think of yourself as a walker, and you find ways to tuck at least 20 minutes of walking into even the busiest day.

By this time, you've pretty thoroughly explored the interesting and convenient walking routes in your area. You know the options—down to the pond; across town to the post office; around the track at the high school—and which route is best suited to the season and the weather. Although on certain days you may have the luxury of driving to a scenic state park and taking your walk there, most of the time you have to make do with the now-familiar walks in your area.

So how do you keep yourself amused for years and years more of walking? The cardinal principle of the Walk It Off! program is that walking is a pleasure and should continue to be a pleasure. In the next chapter I'll discuss ways of increasing the physical challenge of walking. But this chapter focuses

on the mental games you can play to add pleasure to your routine—
and offers some tips for keeping your walking routine from getting
too routine.

Strategies of Veteran Walkers

A neighbor of mine, Helene, was one of my first converts to walking. Helene is the mother of three children under the age of 10.
Although she had registered for, and dropped out of, three consec-
utive aerobic dance classes, she took to walking easily and developed a regular routine in which her husband played with the
children when he arrived home from work, and she ducked out for
a walk.

"What do you do when you're bored with walking?" I asked
her one day in the elevator of our building, after she had been
walking regularly for two years. She laughed, a bit embarrassed,
but proceeded to tell me that she is like Walter Mitty, the meek
James Thurber character who lived in a world of heroic fantasies.

"All day long I'm either surrounded by small children or running somewhere to pick one up from nursery school and drop
another one off at ballet class. I know caring for children is important, but I often feel rather small in the bigger scheme of things.
Other people are staring into microscopes trying to discover a cure
for cancer, or making decisions that affect the destiny of nations,
and I'm picking up toys and wiping runny noses.

"So when I go out to walk," Helene confessed, "I take on the
posture of a world leader. I don't think about my everyday life. I
worry about the labor shortage, interest rates, oil spills, guerrilla
warfare, the situation in the Middle East. And I imagine myself in
a position of power, trying to solve these problems. It's a lot of
fun. And after a couple of months of walking and thinking about
these things, I've actually developed some very strong opinions
about what should be done. I've written a few letters to my con-

gressmen. And now when I'm among adults, my conversation isn't all about the kids.''

Helene has found a personal way to keep walking interesting for herself and to fill a psychological need while she's exercising her body and filling her physiological needs.

Another veteran walker I worked with takes a very different approach. Roger had been a runner for years and enjoyed pushing himself to his physical limits, allowing the strain of exercising to keep all thought of work out of his mind. But he developed a series of stress fractures in his foot, and as I treated him, I tried to persuade him to switch from running to a walking program.

Roger was not an easy patient to convince. Walking didn't feel ''hard'' enough for him; he was sure it wouldn't distract him from thinking about his problems at work. As we talked, I realized that Roger was using exercise as an escape. I suggested that he allow himself to think about work for the first 10 minutes of each walk, and then, when his thoughts began to repeat, consciously switch over to a different walking personality. He could imagine himself running in the Olympics, riding a motorcycle, or dancing in a disco—anything far from his workaday self.

> ''Unhappy businessmen, I am convinced, would increase their happiness more by walking 6 miles every day than by any conceivable change in philosophy,'' said British philosopher Bertrand Russell, who was vigorous and creative until the age of 98.

It was this suggestion that helped Roger become a satisfied walker, although he implemented it in a way that surprised me. ''I'm a party animal,'' he told me with a mischievous grin one day as I was examining his foot. The mental attitude that worked best to keep his mind off work and help him enjoy walking was to think of himself as a carefree teenager. He listened to his Walkman or sang popular rock songs to himself as he walked.

Striking an attitude as you walk can make exercising more fun. It's not necessary to do it in an organized, systematic way, but adopting a walking personality is something you should consider doing at least once in a while. Unlike Helene and Roger, I do not personally have one attitude or mind-set that I don every time I walk. I like variety, and I try to dream up new mental games to play, as well as replaying old favorites.

A game that I find endlessly fascinating to play as I walk involves adopting a "personality of the day." Sometimes I choose a walking personality that expresses my mood. But at other times it's more fun to try on body language that's completely alien to the way I'm feeling—to break through my repetitive thought patterns and introduce a fresh, unfamiliar feeling.

Following are five walking personalities to experiment with. I hope you'll try them all, one walk at a time, to find the ones you enjoy most. As you do, be sure to note which personality you adopted and how it made you feel in your Walker's Log. After a while you'll no doubt make up your own favorite personalities and take them out for a stroll when the mood hits.

The Aggressive Strider

I find this personality easiest to adopt when I'm feeling angry. Imagine yourself a captain of industry, a general leading an army, the commander of a spaceship, or the leader of the A-Team.

You're on a mission. This walk is terribly urgent. Many lives depend on it. Your whole body expresses power and importance as you walk. You gaze forward, undistracted by the sights around you. You hold yourself tall and proud: eyes forward, shoulders back, arms swinging forward in loosely clenched fists. You're super-alert, hurling yourself forward around the track, ready to take on the world. You walk in a punctuated rhythm: *left,* right, *left,* right. You're like a stalking lion. Your motto is "Don't tread on me."

The Sensual Stroller

For this one, think Marilyn Monroe or Elvis Presley. Your whole body is alive with pleasure as you walk. You feel your lithe limbs moving under your clothes. You step forward with a slinky roll, leading with your hips, your arms gracefully flowing forward and back with each sensuous unfolding of your thighs.

You move like a graceful tiger, leisurely but calculating. You're aware of the wind in your hair, the sun on your face. You're beautiful and desirable, and you know it. You're humming something provocative, like "Mama Said There'd Be Days Like This" or "The Girl from Ipanema." You know you look marvelous. You're in the mood for love.

The Rebel Slouch

You're different and you don't care who knows it. You're a majority of one, an unparalleled force, marching to a different drummer. You tie a red bandanna around your head. You sneer like James Dean in *Rebel Without a Cause*. You're not like other people and you don't want to be grouped with them. You have nothing but contempt for the world.

Your posture isn't perfect and you don't care. You're sticking one sneaker out in front of the other, and that had just better be good enough. You take short, jabby steps . . . then shift into long, slouchy ones. You don't have to be consistent.

The great novelist Charles Dickens regularly walked every afternoon for hours at a clip. "If I could not walk far and fast," he wrote, "I think I would just explode and perish."

Your totem is the porcupine, and anyone who bothers you will get stuck. You're humming "Take This Job and Shove It" and your motto is "Who's gonna make me?" or "Don't let the bastards get you down."

The Party Animal

Thank God it's Friday! It's ridiculous how seriously people take themselves and their careers, their checkbooks, their children, their insurance policies. You can't take it with you, so you might as well enjoy it now.

You're playful as a panda bear. You're humming "Seventy-six Trombones" and walking with your chin tilted up, your arms jauntily bent at the elbow, letting your fun side emerge. You're stepping high and fast, and pumping your arms. You gaze eagerly about you, looking for something amusing, something different, something *fun* to concentrate on. You smile at passing children and old people. You grin amiably at yourself in passing store windows. You bark back at dogs. Your motto is "Let the good times roll!"

The Zen Walker

"Be here now" is the slogan of the meditative walker. There's a total awareness of each step taken, each arm movement, each rhythmic breath. Every street sound registers. Each sight is taken in and appreciated. The walk is experienced as a series of moments—each a pearl to be treasured and held up to awareness. When thoughts intrude, they are noted, then gently swept away by concentration on the walk.

Body posture is checked with each step. The roll of the foot on the ground is felt. The body is held gently erect. The sights around you take on a luminous light. You notice particles in the air, the slant of the sun's rays, the shape of the clouds. You lose all sense of yourself and merge with your surroundings.

To preview these walking personalities before you face the outside world, stand in front of a full-length mirror and adopt the aggressive, sensual, rebel, party animal, and Zen postures. We've all read about how body language communicates to other people. But I've noticed that we also communicate to ourselves through the way we carry our bodies on a particular day. Walking is body language in motion. And it's a lot of fun to try to learn some new languages.

Tips for Walking Longevity

To become a lifetime walker, the habit of exercising four or five times a week needs to be continually renewed and refreshed. Although getting into a walking rut is better than being in a no-exercise rut, it's tempting to drop any routine that becomes dull. Here are some ideas on refueling your walking habit and keeping it a meaningful and pleasurable part of your life.

Follow the "perfect-day imperative."

By my count, there are no more than thirty or forty truly lovely days in the average year in New York. I'm talking about those days that have perfect, moderate temperatures and a clear sunny sky. You may have noticed that when these days do occur, they almost never happen on the weekends, when we can spend all day outside enjoying them. But no matter what else is going on in my life, I think it imperative to get out for a walk on every single perfect day. I will cancel lunch dates or postpone work to do it. These perfect days do wonders for renewing my pleasure in walking. My senses open up to my surroundings. My mood soars. And the memories of these walks somehow carry over and help me also get out on the not-so-perfect days that follow.

Declare your independence.

So many of the activities that occupy our days are determined by others. The boss, the customer, the client, the child, the parent, the spouse, the tax collector . . . they all ride herd on us. When I'm walking, I like to think of myself as the Marlboro man without the cigarette—that quintessential American image of personal freedom, the lone pioneering spirit roaming the prairies on his horse.

Many new fitness walkers are women who have traditionally been discouraged from exercising. Or men who have broken away from the jogging, weight-lifting pack to find their own style of exercise. Walkers are an independent, self-sufficient crew. That's something to keep in mind and take pride in.

Don't send yourself negative messages.

It doesn't take much to deflate my ego. One glance at the narrow-hipped beauties in the *Sports Illustrated* bathing suit issue will do it. Or the latest news that caffeine, or radon, or apple pie will damage my body is enough to make me feel not only short, chunky, and unattractive but bound for the hospital. When my self-esteem is low, I use my walks as a kind of psychological make-over. I deliberately count my blessings. As I walk, I go through the affirmations described in Chapter 6. After all, I have good qualities; I enjoy important, caring relationships; I have scored some emotional victories; I've gained some control over my need for fattening foods; and I am a success. Aren't you?

Reidentify your friends, and your enemies.

Some of the people in your life who scoffed at your commitment to walking at first may now be converts themselves. Other early supporters may have become bored with that role and even a bit resentful now that you don't need their help anymore. Look back at Chapter 5 and reevaluate your support systems. If you find they've weakened, it may be time to join a walking club or group and find new support. Perhaps colleagues at work are ready to join you. Sustaining a basic behavior change like walking is one of the hardest things people do; we all need a supportive environment to help us succeed.

Continue to work at building the walking habit.

You may feel that walking has become an ingrained routine and that finding time to walk has become less and less of a problem.

But that doesn't mean you should stop rewarding yourself for doing it! There's something very healthy and reinforcing about trying to dream up ways to reward your walking success. It focuses your thoughts on the things that bring you pleasure and the positive things you can do for yourself. And it keeps walking associated with joy and happiness.

Redefine your goals.

Look back to the walking wish list in Chapter 2, in which you chose your three primary walking goals. Are they still the same? When I began to walk, weight loss and then weight maintenance was my primary walking goal. But today that seems to have subsided in importance. I still put a lot of effort into making sure I eat healthfully and don't gain weight. But that's not my primary challenge. Rather, improving and stabilizing my mood is the chief benefit I seek from walking. Veteran walkers should rethink their goals on occasion. Maybe ''enjoying nature'' now supersedes your earlier goals and you need to reward yourself with some hikes in the country.

15

Walking Plus: Adding Other Exercises

One of the great joys of walking is feeling that even though I'm getting older, I'm improving in physical strength and endurance. I'm certainly more fit and slimmer today than I was ten years ago. That helps me deal with some of the inevitable changes that come with aging (such as gray hairs, or the need for reading glasses) with equanimity and humor. Father Time may score a few points here and there. But walking with a lively step four or five times a week is keeping him at bay.

As you know by now, the Walk It Off! program is not a "get rich quick" scheme. It doesn't result in drastic or instant improvements in fitness. Rather, it's like putting money in a savings account. It doesn't seem like much at first, but little by little it adds up; your strength and endurance grow. And one day, when you're running for a bus or rearranging the living room furniture, you'll find yourself able to draw on reserves of physical prowess you never knew you had.

This happened to me recently on a family skiing trip to

Austria. I'll never be more than an "advanced beginner" on skis. But as I become more fit, skiing does become more enjoyable. In Austria, the slopes were arduous, but I was seldom out of breath. I had no difficulty sidestepping up the mountain to assist my daughters whenever they fell. It felt good to realize how much my strength and stamina had grown because of my disciplined walking regime.

After you have followed the Walk It Off! program for a length of time, you too will one day arrive at an awareness that you're in much better physical condition than you were when you started. If you were overweight and hadn't exercised for years before you began walking, it could take up to two years of walking to condition your muscles, ligaments, and tendons. But whether it happens quickly or slowly, your muscles will eventually respond to regular walking.

What do you do once you've arrived at a state of "fitness"? Should you continue to increase the level of physical challenge? Or should you be content to maintain your gains?

This is a very personal decision. As I mentioned in Chapter 13, a minimal walking program of 20 to 60 minutes four to five times a week is probably all you need to maintain your health, weight, and good mental outlook.

But once you're feeling your oats and enjoying the sense of physical power it's fun to experiment at least with adding additional challenges. And if you're a very goal-oriented person, you may become bored with the walking routine once you can do it easily. It's a good idea to at least *try* adding some other exercises once you're in good condition. You may be surprised to find that exercises you once despised because they overtaxed your body are now easy enough to be fun.

Hitting the Hills

If you live in a hilly area, climbing the hills is a convenient way to extend your walking challenge. As your fitness level improves, you'll find that without getting out of breath you can conquer hills that once made you huff and puff. Hill climbing raises your walking heart rate about 10 to 50 beats a minute. It's an excellent heart conditioner and calorie burner.

> "Listen, it's really quite simple. Walking gives me perspective. To me, the idea that a beautiful grove of trees is like a cathedral is a lot of crap. The cathedral is like a grove of trees. 'Tisn't so much walking, it's what walking puts you in touch with."—COLIN FLETCHER, *The Complete Walker III*

But whatever goes up must come down, and some people find that downhill walking results in knee pain. When you're going downhill, your heel hits the ground with greater force; and since the leg must be more extended at the knee, absorbing the shock of the heel strike can hurt the knee. Good walking shoes can help you avoid pain. But if you have a pair and still get knee pain from downhill walks, try adding a different form of exercise to your walking routine.

Here are some tips for walking on hilly ground:

- Ease into hills by warming up first. Start by walking on level ground. Slow down as you begin climbing uphill, then gradually increase your pace while maintaining comfortable breathing.
- When going up, lean forward, into the hill, and swing your arms vigorously for extra power.

- When going down, lean back slightly and take short, slow steps to reduce the braking impact of each step.
- Cool down by walking on level ground at the end of your walk. To reduce achiness and muscle tightness, be sure to stretch when you get home.

Weights and Packs

Carrying a backpack or hand weights as you walk is a good way to increase the fitness impact and burn more calories. Scientists call this the "overload principle." Physical fitness improves when the body works against loads greater than it normally encounters.

If you take your walks to or from work, you've probably experimented with weights without realizing it. A 7-pound briefcase, a shopping bag, or even a heavy purse adds to your exercise.

Massachusetts governor Michael Dukakis began running in high school and enjoyed the exercise for decades. But at age 50, he admits, "certain joints and parts of my heels began complaining." Governor Dukakis now walks 45 minutes a day with hand weights.

Sports medicine specialists have experimented with increasing the aerobic effect of walking by having walkers add weights to the torso, ankles, wrists, or hands. This does result in an increased energy expenditure. But according to the *Journal of the American Medical Association,* there are potential complications. Systolic blood pressure is increased while exercising with extremity weights. And a number of ankle and wrist injuries have occurred.

You don't *need* weights in order to benefit from the exercise of walking, and you certainly shouldn't walk with weights if doing so makes the activity unpleasant for you. I also strongly advise that people with high blood pressure or cardiac or circulatory problems avoid using weights, which may hike blood pressure even higher. If you have had a back injury or joint problems, weights may exacerbate them by placing extra strain on these places and increasing the likelihood of further injury.

If you have none of these problems, however, and have become an experienced, steady walker, adding weights may add some enjoyment to your program. I use them sometimes when I have only 20 or 30 minutes to walk but I long for a strenuous workout. Weights increase the difficulty—and therefore the aerobic benefit—of walking and let you pack more fitness benefit into shorter workouts.

Here are some tips for using weights properly:

- *Don't* weight yourself all over. Instead, choose one of several weight options, such as wrist weights, a weighted vest, or a weighted belt. If you use a belt, make sure it rests loosely and comfortably on your hips, not tight around your waist.
- *Do* increase the amount of weight you carry very gradually. A general rule is to add no more than 1 pound a week.
- *Don't* allow the weight you carry to exceed 10 percent of your own body weight.
- *Do* consider a backpack or a waist pack ("fanny pack"). These not only increase the difficulty of your walk, but give you an easy, convenient way to carry items you may want to take along, such as sunscreen, bug repellent, keys, money, maps, healthy snacks, and so on.
- *Don't* carry hand weights limply at your sides. To make them work for you, swing your arms to chest or shoulder level to intensify the impact. A recent study showed that when weights are swung vigorously, heart rate increases on an average of 25 beats per minute.

- *Don't* use ankle weights. They can throw off your center of gravity and put too much stress on the knees, causing injuries.

Race Walking

I've seen this walking routine called by dozens of different names, including "striding" and "aerobic," "race," "fitness," "power," "pace," "rhythmic," "health," and "exercise" walking. They all boil down to very similar routines with the same goal: to boost the pace of walking so that your heart rate is kept high during the workout, as it is in running or aerobic dance.

Race walking is a competitive sport with a regulation walking style. It's that funny-looking, hip-twisting walking you see done at the Olympics. One of the things I like best about race walking is that short people, like myself, not only can compete successfully, but actually dominate the sport. Mexico currently has the top race walkers in the world—and they are nowhere near as tall and long-limbed as competitive runners. Still, world-class race walkers cover a mile in less than 6 minutes and the marathon in less than 2:45.

Race walkers burn more calories per mile than runners going at similar speeds. The upper-body and arm movement of race walking produces extra energy expenditure.

Women are finding that race walking is a sport they can compete in successfully. Although it's been an Olympic event since 1908, the upcoming 1992 Summer Olympics will be the first ever to feature a women's race walking event.

There are only two official rules for race walking:

- One foot must be in contact with the ground at all times (otherwise, you are running).
- Your leg must be completely straight as your body passes over it. (This occurs naturally.)

But there are many techniques that help you walk more quickly. If you think you might eventually want to enter competitions (a good idea for the ex-runner who misses the thrill of preparing for marathons), I recommend you take some lessons in technique. The Walker's Club of America and other groups offer courses. There are thousands of race walking competitions around the country— and some are for beginners.

The race walking I suggest in this section is an easier version of the Olympic sport. It differs from the brisk walking of the Walk It Off! program in three ways: pace, heart rate, (or aerobic effect) and posture.

Race walking is generally done at over 3 miles an hour, or 12 to 20 minutes per mile. Brisk walking, on the other hand, can be as slow as 2 miles an hour. Competitive race walkers go at astounding speeds. Contestants in a 50-kilometer (31-mile) race average 7 minutes per mile; the fastest recorded mile was race-walked in under 6 minutes.

Race walking is aerobic. It requires a sustained level of breathing and heart rate. Aerobic activities enable your cardiovascular (heart and blood vessel) system to supply oxygen to your body's major muscle groups so you can do a continuous physical activity. Other aerobic activities include running, swimming, skating, aerobic dancing, and bicycling. Stop-and-start activities, such as football, tennis, and weight lifting, are not aerobic.

The major long-term benefit of aerobic exercise is an overall improvement in your cardiovascular system, which lowers the risk of high blood pressure and heart disease. To gain significant benefits from aerobic actvity, you must do it regularly, from 20 to 60 minutes a session, three to five sessions a week.

Posture during race walking also differs from brisk walking. Because their hips twist, race walkers look very strange to the un-initiated observer, but the modifications from walking fast are actually not as dramatic as they look. It's mostly in the use of the hips and arms. The benefits of race walking include trimming the buttocks and hips and firming the upper torso and arms.

To begin race walking, first practice the following techniques in front of a mirror. Then you'll be less self-conscious when you take it out on the road. Here's how to do it:

Lengthen your stride. To walk faster, you take longer strides—so that you take fewer steps per foot and cover the distance in less time. Measure your pace either in steps per minute or miles per hour, whichever you find easier.

Lead with your arms. An exaggerated arm swing helps you walk faster, propelling your body along. It also helps develop upper-body muscles. And it increases the overall body motion and difficulty of your walk, helping you burn more calories. You can accomplish this in one of two ways. You can swing your arms in very long arcs so that at the top of each arc your arm is high in front of you, almost at shoulder level and parallel to the ground. Or you can bend your elbow at a 90-degree angle and move your arms in a "pumping" motion, with your hands held in loose fists. (Don't clench your fists; that increases the tension in your arms and causes you to hunch up your shoulders, adding an unnatural stiffness to your walking style.) The long arm swing is okay at the beginning, but as your pace increases you may find it awkward. Try to switch to the pumping technique, in which arms stay closer to the body. Many walkers prefer the pumping technique at any speed.

Walk the line. Your feet should land along an imaginary center line that stretches out in front of you. In regular walking, your feet travel along two parallel lines, at the same distance from each other as the width between your feet when you're standing still. But in fitness walking, you bring each foot down directly in front of you so that it lands on the same line the other foot has just left. Because your legs must "swing" around to put your feet in this single line, your hips will pivot slightly, moving from back to front with the step of each corresponding leg. This exaggerated hip movement helps tone your muscles.

Plant your feet. Race walkers concentrate on "planting" their heels at about a 40-degree angle to the ground. The bottom of the foot and the leg should be at a 90-degree angle to each other. As the edge of your heel strikes, tilt your foot very slightly to the outside. Your shoe will become like a rocker, allowing a smooth, speedy transition from heel to toe.

Push off. To accelerate, you pull forward with one leg, pushing straight back with the other until the toe is off the ground. Then swing the other leg forward. This powerful thrusting motion speeds you forward.

Swivel your hips. The hips should be pushed forward as far as possible with each stride to increase the distance covered. This downward and forward extension gives the race walker that distinctive swivel-hipped gait. You might want to practice this component of race walking by attempting to take longer strides.

Time your breathing. Breathing should be deep, even, and rhythmic, keyed to your pace. For maximum speed, coordinate your breathing with your stride. Many race walkers prefer to inhale for two steps, then exhale for two.

Check with your doctor before race walking, especially if you smoke, are over 45, are overweight, or have a history of heart disease, high blood pressure, asthma, diabetes, or foot problems. If your first attempts at race walking leave you feeling breathless or with pain or pressure in your chest, neck, shoulders, or arms, you should see your doctor. He or she may want to give you a stress test to see how your body reacts to aerobic exercise.

Warm-ups and cool-downs are important with any aerobic activity. Walk briskly first, then switch into race walking. And cool down by walking slowly until your heart rate returns to normal. Stopping suddenly will make your heart rate and blood pressure plummet, which is especially dangerous in older walkers.

When you switch to race walking you may experience sore muscles (the doctor may call it "myositis") because you're using different ones than you do in brisk walking. The muscle strain will lessen as you develop muscles in both the front and back of the legs and thighs. Remember to stretch before and after race walking to prevent injury and soreness.

A Mixed Sports Routine

Have you always hated tennis? Felt miserable in aerobic dance class? Been out of breath after just three minutes of jumping rope? Wanted to join the town softball or volleyball team but been afraid of making a fool out of yourself?

There's no guarantee that your regular walking program will change how you feel about other exercises. But it's worth giving them a second chance after your body is conditioned by walking. You may be delighted to find that your early exercise dropout experiences were caused by lack of conditioning, rather than lack of innate ability or desire.

"Leaders of exercise programs often start the participants at too high an intensity and recommend too much exercise," said Dr. Ann Ward, of the University of Massachusetts Medical Center, Worcester, in a round-table discussion on the health benefits of exercise reported in *The Physician and Sportsmedicine*. "We have discouraged people from exercising by making them believe that they have to sweat and reach a certain heart rate, and maybe they don't really want to work that hard.''

Now that you're in good condition from regular walking, you'll be better able to assess the recommendations of exercise teachers and sports coaches. You may find that an exercise you previously rejected as too painful or too hard is now just right.

Veteran walkers find many imaginative ways to alternate walking with other forms of exercise to increase their pleasure and keep themselves interested. Helene, the mother of three young children whom I discussed in Chapter 14, has found that she enjoys walking most in the moderate temperatures of autumn and spring. In the winter she likes to walk only on unusually nice days. So after Christmas each year, as the weather gets nasty, she signs up for a low-impact aerobic exercise class that meets three times a week in the early evening—the time she has set aside as her exercise hour. And during the summer, when she takes her children to a nearby swimming pool every nice day, she swims laps for 30 minutes instead of walking.

An older couple I met while giving a corporate walking class told me they walk all year in order to get in shape for ''spring training'' and take part in a local coed softball team. The husband had played baseball as a boy, but the wife had sat on the sidelines until her 50th birthday. Neither of them is a star player, but after a few years of regular walking they find they can run the bases without a problem and reap tremendous enjoyment from the sport.

Taking the stairs instead of an elevator or escalator is a good way to sneak in some extra exercise and spend some more calories. Several worksite studies have found that people whose only change was using staircases improved their physical fitness by 10 to 15 percent.

Other walkers line up rainy-day alternative exercises. They ride indoor bikes, or use ski or rowing machines. Or they choose to jump rope or do calisthenics or aerobic dance to an exercise video.

Signing up for an intriguing exercise class (tap dancing or karate, ice skating or scuba diving) is another good way to add interest to your walking routine. Groups can be fun as long as you don't waste a lot of mental energy unfavorably comparing yourself to others who may weigh less or be more limber. Now that you're in good condition from walking you'll feel better about yourself and less interested in comparing. The goal of exercise, after all, is not to meet any external standard but simply to approach your "personal best."

16

Preventing Relapses

The Walk It Off! program is deliberately designed to be habit-forming—to create a positive addiction to walking that is associated with pleasure, rewards, and a happy, accepting view of yourself.

But I must be honest with you. Positive addictions are a lot easier to break than are such negative ones as a nicotine, alcohol, drug, or compulsive eating habit. If you don't maintain at least a modest amount of dedication and discipline about walking, your hard-won habit may begin to slip away.

Long-term habit maintenance takes some work. Physicists have developed a concept called "entropy" that I have always found fascinating. Entropy is the natural tendency of things to fall apart. Unless we put some effort into maintaining the walking habit, it's likely to disintegrate from sheer neglect.

Here's how it might happen. You've been walking four times a week, for, say, eighteen months. That extra weight is only a bad memory and your closet is filled with clothes in a new, svelte size. It's natural, at that point, to begin to take success for granted and to focus attention on other parts of your life— your career, perhaps, or your close relationships. Perhaps your mind becomes preoccupied with money problems, redecorating your house, or the health problems of your relatives. You hardly think about walking at all.

If the Walk It Off! exercise and eating program has become a true habit, you're likely to stick with it for many months without even thinking about it. But then, it's almost inevitable that you'll begin to slip. You'll "forget" to walk on some days, or you'll return home after 30 minutes instead of the 60 you've built up to. Your walking shoes will begin to wear out, but you won't replace them. Perhaps you'll also begin to put butter on your bread again, without really noticing the change. Or cookies and potato chips will reappear in your shopping cart. Your pants will start to pinch at the waist, but you won't "notice."

How you respond to these first slips is the key to whether you relapse all the way back to a sedentary, overeating pattern, or recommit yourself to an active, healthy life-style. Maintaining a habit is not as hard as making the major change to begin with—but it is a challenge. It means helping your walking habit survive through slumps, through really bad periods in your life, and through really good ones (falling in love, for instance, or starting an exciting new job) when you're completely distracted.

Over the years, I've gotten into many a "slump" with my walking and eating habits. Sometimes lapses occur because of those famous (and infamous) "circumstances beyond our control." One spring, for example, my two daughters and I consecutively came down with chicken pox, and one daughter followed that up with a bout of pneumonia. For eight weeks running, *someone* in the family was sick. My husband was out of town on business quite a bit during this period, so I had no one to relieve me so I could get out for a walk. I remember that it was snowing outside when the first child got sick. By the time we were all well, temperatures were in the upper 80s. I had entirely missed the brief New York spring.

Because this lapse in my walking habit was truly involuntary, recovery was an easy and joyous process. I couldn't wait to get out in the park and have a few minutes to myself! But I did find I had to walk more slowly for a couple of weeks until I regained my former fitness level. And I had an extra 7 pounds of weight to contend with; it took two months of careful eating to get back into my favorite tight jeans.

More insidious and difficult to deal with is the kind of lapse that occurs for internal reasons. Like most people, I go through periods when I'm less happy than usual. Life seems very bland and routine. Career goals that I've worked hard for don't come through as quickly as I'd hoped. My children seem unruly and troublesome. I don't enjoy being with my friends, and I begin to compare my husband and his all-too-familiar faults with other women's more perfect models. But most devastating, I don't particularly like myself very much. I leaf through the *Sports Illustrated* bathing-suit issue and realize that despite all my healthy eating, my body is not as gorgeous as some. I trudge through my overpacked daily schedule wondering why I'm knocking myself out. I've actually had fantasies about how nice it would be to have a "nervous breakdown" and check into a posh mental institution for a rest.

> Dancer Sandahl Bergman (*A Chorus Line, Dancin', All That Jazz*) began walking with her father after her mother died. At first it was a way to pick up her father's spirits, but she soon realized it was a good workout and she appreciated the low injury rate. "I like it because it's a form of meditation. A time for me to think. And I get fit at the same time."

Mild depression, anger, frustration, and a "blah" view of the universe are at the root of most personal slumps. Staying with the Walk It Off! program during these down periods is probably the best way to shorten them. But it's very easy to feel too discouraged even to go for a walk.

Over the years I've worked out a plan for recovering from slumps in my walking habit and restoring my positive view of myself and the world. The recovery plan involves four steps:

1. recognizing the signs that you're in a slump
2. accepting yourself and your limitations
3. asking for help
4. renewing your commitment to walking

Each step builds on the natural buoyancy of the human spirit. Just as it's normal for us to fall into slumps, it's also normal to bounce back. True, good habits tend to fall apart if left to their own devices. But it's also true that good habits, if carefully cared for, can be maintained and strengthened each time they're successfully reinstated.

1. Recognizing the signs that you're in a slump

Signs of a slump may have nothing directly to do with your exercise or eating patterns at first—which is why slumps are so insidious. The exercise below may give you an early warning.

Are You in a Slump?

Check any statements you currently agree with:

_____ My walking has become irregular.
_____ I'm returning to some of my old eating habits.
_____ I'm sleeping poorly.
_____ I'm losing my temper faster than usual.
_____ I'm taking shorter walks than I used to.
_____ I find myself getting very upset over little things.
_____ I don't look forward to going out for a walk.
_____ I feel I'll never accomplish everything I need to do.
_____ My friends and family members are very irritating.
_____ When I'm tired, food is the first thing I think about.
_____ I don't really "give a damn."
_____ My lack of discipline keeps me a failure.
_____ I'd like to run away from my life.
_____ I'm not happy with the way I look.
_____ Walking is not really worth the effort.

_____ My life feels meaningless these days.
_____ I'm afraid I will never exercise and always be fat.
_____ I don't have much to look forward to.
_____ People seem bent on annoying me.
_____ My schedule is overwhelming.

If you checked only one or two of the above statements you're probably not in a real slump, though you have some symptoms. Go back and look at the statements you checked and resolve to do something about them. If you stop your slump early, you'll have a much easier time recommitting yourself to walking.

If you checked more than two of the above statements, you may already be in a slump. Consider this an emergency situation. You didn't work long and hard at building a walking habit to let it slip away without a good fight. Proceed to the next step.

2. Accepting yourself and your limitations

When you see warning signs of relapse, find some way to express how you feel. You might write yourself a letter, keep a journal, talk into a tape recorder, or simply talk to yourself out loud while you're taking a shower. Some people can express themselves best through dancing, painting, playing the guitar, or singing the blues. Whatever method you choose, provide an escape hatch for the negative tide. Don't try to bury it, ignore it, or keep it bottled up inside.

Once you've expressed your negative feelings you can try to figure out what's behind them. It's often hard to trace the genesis of a funk once you're in it. But I've found that an unaccepting perfectionism is often behind the slumps that veteran walkers get into. To me, it happens something like this. One weekend I overeat and on Monday morning my skirt doesn't fit the way I'd like. I feel very defeated and negative about myself. What's the use of going for my morning walk? It won't immediately undo the damage. And it's obvious I don't have the strength of character to eat the way I know I should.

"A sedentary life is the real sin against the Holy Spirit. Only those thoughts that come by walking have any value."—FRIEDRICH NIETZSCHE, *Maxims and Missiles*

This kind of perfectionism can snowball into a genuine relapse if you let it. The idea that a few slips make you a total failure is widespread in our society, which often encourages us to think unrealistically about what human beings are capable of. I have great respect for the Alcoholics Anonymous and Overeaters Anonymous programs. But I disagree heartily with them in one respect: I don't believe that a few slips mean you are back to day one in changing your habits. In fact, this perfectionist attitude can itself cause relapses. You think: "I didn't walk at all last week, so what the hell, I might as well give up entirely."

A much healthier attitude—and one that can help you succeed in the long run—is to accept the fact that you will slip up on occasion. "The belief that a slip means you have no willpower or are addicted is a self-fulfilling prophecy. If you think it is so, then you act that way," psychologist Dr. G. Allen Marlatt of the University of Washington told the *New York Times*. "A slip is an error in learning, not a failure in willpower." Successful walkers treat the slip as a mistake they need not repeat. And as they recover from the slip, this knowledge gives them confidence in their ability to resist later temptation.

After you've given yourself a little lecture on perfectionism, take a look at your Walker's Log and review your positive accomplishments. Remember that you'll never "go back" to what you were. You're already past that. You've already had the positive experience of walking and have learned a lot about yourself.

Here are some positive thoughts I use to replace negative, perfectionist thinking:

- It's normal to slip up on occasion.
- Even though I've slipped, I can recover my balance.

- I can learn from each lapse and avoid similar ones in the future.
- I've already accomplished a lot of regular walking and healthy eating.
- I can get back on track again and regain my confidence.

3. Asking for Help

Once you're viewing your slump as a temporary state rather than a permanent failure, you need a strategy for pulling out of it. If you catch the slump early, simply reviewing what you know about habit building, reassessing your current walking goals, and reinstating the reward process may be all it takes to recover your momentum.

But if you've tried to renew yourself and failed, it's essential that you seek help. Go back to Chapter 2 and reanalyze your support systems. Whom can you confide in about your lapses in walking? Whom can you count on to encourage you to get back on track?

When I'm in a slump I try to talk to at least three different people about it. The first one is always the hardest. After all, I've been on television talking about walking, I've lectured corporate audiences and taught at health spas. How embarrassing to admit that I sometimes have trouble following my own advice!

Choose the most reliably helpful person you know as your first confessor. Simply tell the truth: I'm in a slump; I haven't walked for several days now; I'm having trouble sticking to my healthy plan; I don't feel very good about myself.

" 'Will you walk a little faster?' said a whiting to a snail.
" 'There's a porpoise close behind us, and he's treading on my tail.' "—LEWIS CARROLL, *Alice's Adventures in Wonderland*

Then listen very carefully to your friend's response. I sometimes even take notes, because I know that when I'm in a bad mental state I ignore positive statements. A friend may say, "Well, you may have gained a couple of pounds, but it doesn't show. You still look okay. You're always happier when you're walking than when you're not. Is there something I can do to help?''

Don't brush aside compliments. Take them in! Accept the good news about yourself. And accept all offers of help. Yes, you would like your friend to come along with you for a walk that day. Yes, it would help if you could eat a soup-and-salad lunch together at the local coffee shop. Yes, you will come along with her on a joint shopping trip to buy new walking shoes.

There's no need to feel guilty about accepting such help. Think back to the times when you've helped other people. It made you feel good, didn't it? So accept help when you need it and allow your friends the pleasure of helping.

In order not to lean too heavily on any one person when I'm in a slump, I go on to tell my troubles to at least two others. And each time I try to listen very carefully to the offered advice and let it penetrate my gloomy state. I accept all compliments with a simple ''Thank you,'' and even write them down so I can remember them later. And I accept all offers of help.

Fortified by my friends, I turn back to my family group for additional help. Sometimes I say something like ''Kids, Mommy needs help. I'm under a lot of pressure. You can help by getting your own breakfast in the morning so I can get out and start walking again.'' Or I ask my husband to take over some of my usual household tasks, like paying the bills, or cleaning up after dinner, so I can get to bed very early for a few days and recover my sense of balance.

Sometimes I also seek support and help from walking clubs. I'll attend a lecture on the benefits of walking, or go out on a charity walk and just let the enthusiasm of other people ignite my own.

4: Renewing your commitment to walking

When you first started the Walk It Off! program you took some time to think about yourself, your past exercise experiences, the things that made you happy, and the goals you wanted to accomplish. Although it's not necessary to repeat this process to pull yourself out of a slump, it is necessary to refocus on yourself.

When I'm in a slump I notice that I often worry more about my husband's and children's exercise habits than my own. In an attempt to avoid looking at myself, I focus on how they're feeling.

To get out of a slump, it's necessary to take a "time-out" for yourself. The ideal solution is to take a vacation somewhere that invites walking—a week at the beach or in a national park makes regaining the walking habit a joy.

If that's impossible, perhaps you can get away for a weekend visit to friends or relatives. Let them know that you need to rest and spend some time alone, so they don't arrange a busy schedule for you.

At the very least, take a day off for yourself. Arrange for a baby-sitter to take the children and spend the day in bed napping, resting, and reading. Or get out in the country or a park for the day, with a blanket to rest on, a nice lunch, and a portable radio.

During your time-out, your main goal is to be kind to yourself. Treat yourself as you would a good friend: with sympathy and understanding. Give yourself some compliments. Remember you have:

- good qualities
- important, caring relationships
- control over negative habits
- some emotional victories
- successful accomplishments

Review the positive things that walking has meant in your life. Remember how it's helped you feel physically energized, kept your weight steady, and improved your self-image. Remember the delights of seeing the first green leaves unfurling as you walked in the woods in early spring. Or the feeling of accomplishment of making it eight times around the 1/2-mile track at the high school.

You may not be able to recapture those feelings immediately. But you can certainly *act as if* you're really enjoying your walk. You can smile and make pleasant comments to yourself and others.

When you restart the Walk It Off! program, do it at a slightly easier level than you were at before you began to slump. Go back to the intermediate or even the beginner's routine. Commit yourself to walking 20 minutes, four times a week, even if you were up to 60 minutes at one point. Ease yourself back into the walking habit.

To keep your spirit up, be sure to enter all your walks into your Walker's Log and to reward yourself with a ''me break'' each and every time you walk. If you've gained weight as well as lost momentum in walking, don't try to recover both at the same time. Get back into the walking habit first, and then, a few weeks later, use your renewed confidence to return to a healthier eating pattern.

Recovering from a slump and returning to enthusiastic walking is one of the most powerful things you can do to strengthen your positive addiction. You'll gain insight into the external and internal pressures that can throw you into a slump, and you can learn to head off slumps before they occur. Remember, a broken arm often mends stronger than it was originally.

I've found that holiday periods are when I'm most likely to go into a walking slump. I'm super-busy with preparing for company, shopping for food, cooking, getting the family's good clothes in order, buying gifts, and trying to keep my podiatry practice running when my staff is also preoccupied with holiday preparations. Then there's the tension of large groups of relatives descending on my home, the emphasis on eating, and my desire that my family and my home make a great impression on everyone.

It's very easy to let my dedication to walking, eating healthfully, and taking some time for myself slip during this period. But recently I've found a way to avoid the holiday slump. When my house is full of company, I make a group walk to the park part of the holiday agenda. If possible, I schedule a walk between the dinner and the dessert course. My guests were a bit wary at first, but they've grown used to bringing along a pair of sneakers when they come to visit. It's really fun to get three generations out in the park together. The children run around and release some of their pent-up energy. The adults mingle, talk, and work off a few calories. Soon we're all in a better mood and better able to enjoy one another.

Periods of overwork are another danger point I've identified. If I'm physically and emotionally exhausted, it's very difficult to "do the right thing" for my body and mind. When I approach this point, I immediately ask for help from family and friends. It's amazing how willing people are to pitch in when you ask them! And with their help, I'm able to cut back on my commitments, take some time off to rest and think, and get myself happily back into walking.

When you successfully recover from a slump and have again been walking regularly for a few weeks, dream up a wonderful milestone celebration for yourself. Browse through your Walker's Log to review your accomplishments. Compliment yourself. And take at least a day to do something pleasurable for yourself. As a walker, you deserve all the help and praise you can get from others. But you also need to be your own best friend. A lifelong walking habit, maintained through good times and bad, is the best way there is to keep up a healthy, productive, and happy relationship with yourself.

Happy walking!

Preventing Relapses—in a Nutshell

- Note the signs of a slip: irregular walking, overeating, negative thinking, bad moods.
- Express your feelings.
- Accept the human tendency to slip up.
- Review your previous walking accomplishments.
- Practice positive thinking.
- Ask for help.
- Take some time out for yourself.

- Renew your commitment to walking.
- Start walking at an easier level than before.
- Give yourself some compliments.
- Enter all walks in your Walker's Log.
- Reward yourself with a "me break" for each walk.
- Review the circumstances that led to the lapse and devise preventive strategies for the future.
- When you're back on track, give yourself a milestone reward.

The Walker's Log

Why keep a log? Keeping a record of my walks has been very important in enabling me to keep to the program. For me, it's important to measure my accomplishments. I agree with the sign that Albert Einstein kept in his study: "Not everything that's important can be counted, and not everything that can be counted is important." But so many other things in my life are countable: the dollars I earn, the number of patients I see, the number of hours I work. And these things seem to take on an inflated importance simply because they are measurable quantities of "success." So one way to emphasize to myself the very real importance of walking is to keep track of the number of times I do it. I then have something in print to remind me of my accomplishments. And, embarrassing as it is to admit, I really enjoy flipping back over the pages of my log and reviewing my success at sticking to an exercise program. Since I give myself a milestone reward at the end of every month in which I have walked sixteen or more times, looking at the log also has some pleasant associations.

Another reason for keeping a log is to keep track of the effect walking has on my mood. When I'm feeling irritable or upset, its easy for me to assume that the problem is coming from outside myself—from the daily hassles of life, or from other people. My log reminds me that the mood is at least in part physiological. The hassles don't go away, nor do the other people, but after a walk I'm much better able to cope with them.

Here are some sample pages from my recent Walker's Log to give you an idea how to keep your own.

MONTH: *October*
Day: Monday
Date: 1
Time Walked: 7:30 a.m.; 30 minutes
Miles Walked: 2
Terrain or Route: Flat terrain; Central Park Reservoir
Weather: Sunny, breezy
Mood Before: Sleepy
Mood After: Peaceful, calm
Notes: Saw unusual warbler, migrating south?

Day: Tuesday
Date: 2
Time Walked: 8 a.m.; 45 minutes
Miles Walked: 3
Terrain or Route: Flat terrain; Central Park Reservoir
Weather: Cloudy, cool
Mood Before: Angry; hassle with children over eating breakfast
Mood After: Amused
Notes: Chatted with a neighbor who was also walking.

Day: Wednesday
Date: 3
Time Walked:
Miles Walked:
Terrain or Route:
Weather: Pounding rain; decided to skip walk.
Mood Before:
Mood After:
Notes:

Day: Thursday
Date: 4
Time Walked: 12 p.m.; 30 minutes

Miles Walked: 2¼
Terrain or Route: Flat terrain; wove from Madison to Fifth Avenue, up to 59th Street and back.
Weather: Rain stopped midmorning
Mood Before: Tense, frustrated
Mood After: Very happy
Notes: Good to get out as soon as rain stopped; felt cooped up in office; came back in excellent mood and went through piles of work in the afternoon.

Day: Friday
Date: 5
Time Walked: 8:30 a.m.; 60 minutes
Miles Walked: 4¼
Terrain or Route: Hilly; new path in Central Park
Weather: Cold, sunny
Mood Before: Neutral
Mood After: Peaceful, relaxed
Notes: Felt strong enough for an extended workout.

Day: Saturday
Date: 6
Time Walked: 2 p.m.; 30 minutes
Miles Walked: 2
Terrain or Route: wove from Madison to Fifth Avenue to 79th Street and back.
Weather: Partly sunny; brisk
Mood Before: Lonely
Mood After: Happy
Notes: Convinced Bart to go with me.

Day: Sunday
Date:
Time Walked:
Miles Walked:
Terrain or Route:
Weather: Drizzly, cool
Mood Before:
Mood After:
Notes: Took day off; did some stretching in house.

MONTH	DAY	DATE	TIME WALKED	MILES WALKED	TERRAIN OR ROUTE

WEATHER	MOOD BEFORE	MOOD AFTER	NOTES